PRAISE FOR CATHY GLASS

'Poignant and revealing ... [the] ... se have helped to move and insp... ...ion' *Sunday Mirror*

'A true tale of hope' *OK!* Magazine

'Heartbreaking' *Mirror*

'A life-affirming read ... that proves sometimes a little hope is all you need' *Heat* Magazine

'A hugely touching and emotional true tale' *Star* Magazine

'Foster carers rarely get the praise they deserve, but Cathy Glass's book should change all that' *First* Magazine

'Cannot fail to move those who read it' *Adoption-net*

'Once again, Cathy Glass has blown me away with a poignant story' The Writing Garnet, book blogger

'Brilliant book. I'd expect nothing less from Cathy ... I cried, of course' Goodreads review

'... gripping page-turner from start to finish ... emotive and heart-wrenching ...' Kate Hall, book blogger

Too Scared
to Tell

ALSO BY CATHY GLASS

FOSTERING MEMOIRS
Cut
The Silent Cry
Daddy's Little Princess
Nobody's Son
Cruel to be Kind
The Night the Angels Came
A Long Way from Home
A Baby's Cry
The Saddest Girl in the World
Please Don't Take My Baby
Will You Love Me?
I Miss Mummy
Saving Danny
Girl Alone
Where Has Mummy Gone?
Damaged
Hidden
Mummy Told Me Not to Tell
Another Forgotten Child
The Child Bride
Can I Let You Go?
Finding Stevie
Innocent

INSPIRED BY HER OWN EXPERIENCES
The Girl in the Mirror
My Dad's a Policeman
Run, Mummy, Run

SHARING HER EXPERTISE
Happy Kids
Happy Adults
Happy Mealtimes for Kids
About Writing and How to Publish

WRITING AS LISA STONE
The Darkness Within
Stalker
The Doctor

THE MILLION COPY BESTSELLING AUTHOR

CATHY GLASS

Too Scared to Tell

**Abused and alone, Oskar has no one.
A true story.**

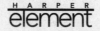

Certain details in this story, including names, places and dates, have been changed to protect the family's privacy.

HarperElement
An imprint of HarperCollins*Publishers*
1 London Bridge Street
London SE1 9GF

www.harpercollins.co.uk

HarperCollins*Publishers*
1st Floor, Watemarque Building, Ringsend Road
Dublin 4, Ireland

First published by HarperElement 2020

9 10 8

A catalogue record of this book is available from the British Library

ISBN 978-0-00-838038-0

Printed and bound in Great Britain by
CPI Group (UK) Ltd, Croydon

MIX
Paper from
responsible sources
FSC™ C007454

This book is produced from independently certified FSC™ paper to ensure responsible forest management.

For more information visit: www.harpercollins.co.uk/green

ACKNOWLEDGEMENTS

A big thank-you to my family; my editors, Carolyn and Holly; my literary agent, Andrew; my UK publishers HarperCollins, and my overseas publishers, who are now too numerous to list by name. Last, but definitely not least, a big thank-you to my readers for your unfailing support and kind words. They are much appreciated.

A third of children who have
been sexually abused never tell.

CHAPTER ONE

BEING WATCHED

'I feel dreadful,' the young teacher wept. 'His uncle is angry with me, Oskar is sobbing, and now he has to live with a strange family.'

'It might not be for long,' I said. 'Just until his mother gets back. And we're not that strange,' I added, trying to lighten her mood.

'No, I didn't mean that,' she said, forcing a small smile through her tears. 'I'm sure you're very nice, but it's not Oskar's home, is it?'

'I'll do my best to make it home while he is with me,' I said, touching her arm reassuringly. Erica Jordan, Oskar's teacher, was blaming herself for Oskar coming into foster care. 'It wasn't your decision to bring Oskar into care,' I pointed out.

'No, but I logged everything he told me and reported it to my Headmistress.'

'Which was right,' I said. 'That was the correct procedure. If you hadn't reported your concerns and something dreadful had happened to Oskar, how would you have felt then?'

'I'd never have forgiven myself. I'm sorry,' she said, wiping her eyes. 'I'm only in my second year of teaching and I've never dealt with anything like this before.'

'I understand, and believe me, it doesn't matter how experienced you are, it's still upsetting. No one wants to see a child removed from their home, but sometimes it's necessary to keep them safe.'

'I don't think Oskar has much of a home from what he's told me,' she admitted.

'No, but the social services will thoroughly investigate. I've been a foster carer for a long time, and a child who regularly arrives at school unkempt and so hungry that he has to steal food – as Oskar has – suggests they are not being looked after at home. It doesn't mean he'll remain in care for good, just until the social services are satisfied that if he goes home he'll be properly cared for.'

Being hungry and unkempt weren't the only reasons Oskar, aged six, was being brought into care. He was pale, withdrawn and so tired he kept falling asleep in class, and sometimes he arrived at school with unexplained bruises on his arms and legs. He had first come to the school in January, so four months previously, and the concerns had been there right from the start, which Miss Jordan had been correctly reporting to the Headmistress. Although Oskar's mother had first registered him at the school, a series of 'uncles' had been bringing and collecting him, sometimes arriving very late. Originally from Eastern Europe, Oskar and his mother had good English, but the uncles claimed to have none.

Miss Jordan had also told me that the school had set up a number of meetings with his family to try to discuss their concerns, but no one had ever turned up. Now, on the second day back at school after the Easter holidays, Oskar had arrived very late, hungry, in tears and with an angry red mark on his face. The man who had dropped him off at the entrance to the school had gone straight away, when those arriving late were expected to bring the child into the school and sign them in. Now even more concerned for the boy's welfare, the Headmistress had asked Miss Jordan, who had established a relationship with Oskar, to talk to him privately, one to one, to try to find out as much as possible, while she contacted the social services again. Reluctant at first to say anything about his home, Oskar finally told her his mother had been away for most of the two-week holiday and his uncles had been left in charge of him. He said the mark on his cheek was from one of his uncles, who had slapped him that morning for not doing as he was told. The social services had tried to contact his mother without success, so, not wanting Oskar to return home, they had applied to the court for an emergency protection order to bring him into care temporarily. At the same time, I'd received a phone call from my supervising social worker, Edith, putting me on standby to receive Oskar if the court order was granted. Edith had phoned again at midday to say the order had been granted and I should go to Oskar's school at three o'clock to collect him.

It was now nearly 4.15 p.m. and most of the other children had gone home. I was with Miss Jordan in her classroom while Oskar, his social worker, the Headmistress and the uncle who'd arrived to collect him were in another room. Also with them was a teaching assistant who worked at the school and was now acting as an impromptu translator for the uncle. It was pure luck she spoke his language, having come to the UK from the same country many years before. I'd said goodbye to my previous foster children, Molly and Kit, in very unhappy circumstances a few days before. (I tell their story in *Innocent*.) Aware that foster carers are in short supply and my spare room never stayed empty for long, I'd given it a thorough clean and prepared it for the next child virtually straight away.

It's a strange feeling when a child or children you've loved and cared for leave, like a mini bereavement. But as a foster carer you have to be brave and stoical and remind yourself you have done your best and that the children are now able to return home or go to a loving adoptive family so they can move on with their lives. While each child comes with a different story, one thing they all have in common is that they need loads of love, understanding, kindness and reassurance. The last of which Miss Jordan needed too.

She seemed a bit happier now I'd told her that Oskar's social worker was sure to arrange contact so he could see his mother. As we talked, waiting for his social worker to finish the meeting in the room next door, my mobile rang. It was Edith, my supervising social worker. 'I'd better take this,' I said to Miss Jordan.

'Yes, of course.'

'Have you got Oskar yet?' Edith asked.

'I'm at his school now. His social worker is with him. Shall I call you once I'm home?'

'Yes. Leave a voicemail message if I don't pick up and I'll speak to you tomorrow.'

'OK.' Sometimes Edith updated me, but more often I updated her. As a supervising social worker (SSW) her role was to monitor, support, advise and guide the foster carers she was responsible for in all aspects of fostering.

Just as I ended the call and returned my phone to my bag, the classroom door opened and a tallish man in his thirties with fair hair came in with a small boy beside him.

'Oskar, love,' Miss Jordan said, immediately standing and going to him.

I went over too.

'I'm Andrew Holmes, Oskar's social worker,' the man said to me. He must have already met Erica Jordan.

'Cathy Glass, foster carer,' I said, smiling at Oskar.

'This is the lady I told you about,' Andrew explained to him.

'Hello, Oskar,' I said gently, my heart going out to him. He was pale, slightly built, small for his age and his eyes were red from crying. He looked at me, petrified. The bruise on his cheek was even more pronounced against his pallid skin.

'Are you OK, Oskar?' Miss Jordan asked, squatting down in front of him so she was at his height. He gave a small nod, wide-eyed and anxious.

'Cathy is going to look after you for a few days until your mummy gets back,' she said, which wasn't strictly true and made it sound as though he would automatically be returned to his mother when she reappeared. I knew Miss Jordan was trying her best to comfort him, but I'd learnt from years of fostering that we have to be careful what we tell children and not give them false hope.

'I'll see you tomorrow,' she said to him, straightening.

'Will Oskar be coming to school tomorrow?' I checked with his social worker. It was usual for a child to go to school the day after coming into care, as it offered some routine and familiarity.

'Yes. I don't see why not,' Andrew replied.

'You'll see your teacher in the morning,' I told Oskar, with another reassuring smile. He stared back at me, lost and bewildered.

'Mr Nowak, the man who came to collect Oskar, says he is able to contact Oskar's mother,' Andrew said to me and Miss Jordan. 'He's going to call her and ask her to phone me. Once

I've spoken to her, I'll have a better understanding of what the situation is at home.'

'Will Oskar be seeing his uncles?' I asked. I needed to know in case one of them approached me at the school gates.

'Not until I've spoken to his mother and got a clearer picture of the set-up at home,' Andrew said. 'As far as I can tell, none of the "uncles" is related to Oskar and no one – apart from his mother – is responsible for him.'

That in itself was worrying and was news to Miss Jordan. 'I had assumed they were real uncles,' she said, obviously concerned. 'I'm sure that's what his mother said when she first registered him.'

Andrew gave a non-committal nod, then said to me, 'I'll try to get some of Oskar's clothes, but at present he's just got what he's wearing.' This isn't unusual. More often than not, if it's an emergency placement, the child arrives with what they have on.

'I've got plenty of spares,' I said.

'His coat is here,' Miss Jordan said, and she crossed the classroom to fetch it from a peg.

'Am I going now?' Oskar asked in a small voice.

'Yes, shortly,' Andrew said. Then to me, 'I'll let you have the placement forms as soon as they're ready.' These usually came ahead of the child or with them if the placement was planned in advance, but as this was an emergency there hadn't been time. 'As far as Mr Nowak is aware, Oskar hasn't got any allergies and there are no special dietary or cultural needs,' he added. This type of information would have been included in the placement forms. 'Hopefully I'll know more once I've spoken to Oskar's mother.'

'All right,' I said. Having so little information wasn't unheard of, but it was worrying, as I could easily miss something vital while looking after Oskar. 'He's not on any medication? Inhalers for asthma?' I asked.

'Not as far as we know,' Andrew replied.

'None has been brought into school,' Miss Jordan confirmed as she helped Oskar into his coat.

'Are you my mummy now?' Oskar asked his teacher, his bottom lip trembling. Immediately she teared up.

'Miss Jordan is your teacher,' I said gently. 'I'm your foster carer. I'm going to look after you for a while in my house. It's a short ride in my car. You'll have your own bedroom and my grown-up children will help you too. We also have a cat. Do you like cats?'

He gave a small nod.

'Great. I know he's going to like you.'

'I'll phone you tomorrow,' Andrew said to me.

I said goodbye to him and Miss Jordan, and Oskar and I left the classroom. I was still holding his hand and kept talking to him positively as we made our way out of the school. Bless him – six years old, and only in the country a few months, and he was now coming to live with me in a 'strange house', as Miss Jordan had put it. I felt his hand tighten in mine. Although I was doing my best to comfort and reassure him, I knew how lost and alone he must feel.

It was now 4.30 p.m. and, in April, still light outside. We continued along the pavement towards my car. Other vehicles were parked along the kerb and as we approached my car Oskar suddenly stopped and looked across the road. I followed his line of vision and saw a black car parked directly opposite mine. I could see two men sitting in the front and both appeared to be watching us. 'Do you know those men?' I asked as I unlocked my car.

He didn't reply but was still frozen to the spot, staring at the car and looking worried. 'Oskar, get in the car, love,' I said, opening the rear door.

In silence, he did as I asked. I leant in and fastened his seat-belt. He was craning his neck to look at the black car. I closed his car door, then went round and got into the driver's seat. As I did, I glanced over again. Now they were studying me.

'Do you know those men?' I asked Oskar again, turning in my seat to look at him.

'No,' he said, but I could tell from his expression that he did and also that he was worried, if not scared, by their presence.

'You're safe with me,' I said, but before I started the engine I pressed the central locking system, so none of the doors could be opened from the outside. I wasn't being paranoid; I had no idea who those men were, why they were taking such an interest in us or why Oskar should be frightened of them. Had he come from a large extended family, I might have thought they were part of his family and wanted to see where he was being taken. It had happened to me before, just as it's happened to other carers: a child is placed, the carer's address is purposely withheld and then a family member follows the foster carer home on the school run. However, as far as I knew at that point, Oskar only had his mother, and she wasn't in the country. Perhaps they were some of Oskar's 'uncles', but then why had he denied knowing them? I couldn't begin to guess who they were.

As I pulled away the car remained where it was. Even so, I glanced in my rear-view mirror every so often just to check we weren't being followed home. There was no sign of the car.

I talked to Oskar as I drove, telling him about my family and reassuring him there was nothing to worry about. He sat very quiet and still, mainly gazing out of his side window. It was impossible to know what he was thinking or feeling. From the few words he'd spoken, his English seemed to be very good – surprisingly good, considering he'd only been in the country a few months. We arrived home just before 5.00 p.m. and as I parked outside my house I asked him one more time: 'Do you have any idea who those men were?'

'No.'

So I let the matter drop. What I didn't know at the time was that I was going to have to return to the subject very soon.

CHAPTER TWO

ANXIOUS

Only my youngest daughter Paula, twenty-one, was at home when I arrived with Oskar. She was studying for a business degree at a local college and was often in ahead of my other two children – Adrian, twenty-five, and Lucy, twenty-three – who both worked. As soon as Paula heard my key in the front door, she was in the hall ready to greet us.

'I got your text, Mum. Hi, Oskar,' she said brightly. We had a family WhatsApp group so my children and I could message each other collectively. It had largely replaced leaving notes. I'd texted our group earlier to let them know Oskar was coming to stay with us. Having grown up with fostering, my family were used to children and young people suddenly arriving.

'This is my daughter, Paula,' I told Oskar as I helped him out of his coat. He looked at Paula with the same mixture of angst and bewilderment as he had when looking at me.

'Nice to meet you, Oskar,' Paula said, smiling at him.

'He's a little quiet at present,' I told her when he didn't respond.

'That's OK, he'll get used to us.' She threw him another reassuring smile.

At that point Sammy, our rescue cat, strutted into the hall to see who had invaded his territory. He'd been a bit feral when we'd first had him but could now be relied upon not to eat the children.

'Your cat,' Oskar said, staring at the cat.

'Yes, he's called Sammy,' I said. 'Would you like to stroke him?'

He was showing the same reluctance to greet Sammy as Sammy was to him. Paula picked up the cat and presented him to Oskar. He tentatively stroked him.

'Sammy likes you,' Paula said, and finally Oskar's expression gave way to a tiny smile. I breathed a sigh of relief.

Oskar stroked Sammy a few more times and then our cat, a little short on patience, jumped from Paula's arms and disappeared down the hall. Oskar looked after him but didn't try to follow him as another child might.

'Let's take off your shoes,' I said, undoing the Velcro. I helped him out of his shoes and left them with ours in the hall. His shoes, like his clothes, were in poor condition, as were those of many of the children I'd fostered.

Before I'd left home to collect Oskar from school, I'd set out some toy boxes in the living room ready for our return. I'd found that playing can often distract a child from their worries and help them to feel at home and start to relax.

'Let's go and find some toys,' I said enthusiastically. 'Would you like a snack first to see you through till dinner?'

He shook his head, so taking his hand we went into the living room. It's at the back of the house with large glass patio doors that overlook the garden.

'Would you like to play?' Paula asked encouragingly, going over to the toy boxes.

Oskar looked at them and then at me. 'Where do I have to sleep?' he asked anxiously.

'You have your own bedroom upstairs,' I said. 'It's not bedtime yet, but would you like to see your room now?'

He nodded.

'That's fine,' I said. 'This way.' It was slightly unusual for a child of his age to be more interested in their bedroom than toys. Teenagers can't wait to chill out in their own rooms, but not so with younger children.

'Shall I put dinner on?' Paula asked. 'I'm hungry.'

'Yes, please. There's a casserole in the fridge that just needs popping in the oven.'

While Paula went to the kitchen, I took Oskar upstairs. Children react differently to the stress of coming into care: some are very loud and display challenging behaviour, while others, like Oskar, are quiet and withdrawn. The latter is more worrying, as it suggests the child is internalizing their pain, rather than letting it out.

'There's nothing to worry about,' I told him as we followed the landing round to his bedroom. He was holding my hand – in fact, gripping it quite tightly. 'Do you have your own bedroom at home?' I asked him as his gaze travelled warily around his room. He looked at me, confused. 'Or do you share a bedroom?' Information like this would usually have been available on the placement forms, had the move been planned in advance. It would have helped me build up a picture of Oskar's home life before coming into care so I could better meet his needs; for example, if a child is used to sharing a bedroom with siblings, they might need a lot of reassurance on their first few nights of sleeping alone.

'I sleep with Mummy,' Oskar said.

'OK.' Although I wouldn't have expected a child of Oskar's age to be sleeping with a parent.

'And Maria, Elana and Alina,' he added.

'Who are they?' I asked, puzzled.

He shrugged.

'Are they your sisters?'

He shook his head.

'Cousins? Friends?'

He shrugged again and began to look very worried, so I didn't pursue it. Perhaps he was just confused by all the changes, but I'd have to tell his social worker. He would be checking Oskar's home and seeing the sleeping arrangements for himself before he returned Oskar to his mother's care.

'We've got a nice big garden,' I said, drawing him to the window. His room was at the rear of the house and overlooked the garden. He was just tall enough to see over the windowsill. 'You can play out there when the weather is nice, and we also have a park nearby.'

Oskar turned from the window to survey the room. 'Do you like your bedroom?' I asked. He didn't reply. 'Once we have some of your belongings from home in here it will feel more comfortable.' Still no response. 'Would you like to see the rest of the upstairs?'

He gave a small nod.

He slipped his hand into mine again and I showed him the toilet first, and at the same time asked him if he needed to use it, but he didn't. 'This is Adrian's room,' I said, moving to the next door along the landing. 'He's grown up now, but you'll meet him later when he gets in from work.' I opened Adrian's bedroom door just so Oskar could see inside. 'All our bedrooms are private,' I said. 'Just for us.' I closed Adrian's door and went along the landing, opening and closing

13

the girls' bedroom doors, the bathroom and finally my bedroom.

'There is where I sleep,' I said.

He looked in. 'Do I sleep in here?'

'No, love, in your own bedroom, the one we went in first. If you need me in the night, just call out and I'll come to you.'

He looked puzzled and then asked, 'Do you sleep by yourself?'

'Yes. I'm divorced. Do you know what that means?'

He nodded. 'Mummy is.'

'OK. Come on, let's find something to do,' I said, and closed my bedroom door.

'Shall I go to bed?' he asked.

'It's a bit early yet. Come downstairs with me and you can play, then we'll have dinner, and later you can go to bed.'

Oskar did as I asked, and once we were downstairs he came with me into the kitchen-diner where Paula was laying the table ready for dinner later. 'Thanks, love,' I said to her.

'I need to get on with some college work now,' she said.

'Yes, you go. Thanks for your help.'

'I'll see you at dinner,' she told Oskar and, with a smile, left.

The casserole was cooking in the oven and wouldn't be ready for half an hour, so I suggested to Oskar that we go into the living room and play with some toys. He came with me, obedient and compliant but not enthusiastic. We sat on the floor by the toy boxes and I began taking out some of the toys, games and puzzles, trying to capture his interest. He watched me but didn't join in. I wasn't wholly surprised. It might take days, if not weeks, before he relaxed enough to play. Children vary.

14

'Do you understand why you are in care and staying with me for now?' I asked him. Although his social worker would have explained this and I had talked to Oskar about it in the car, there was so much to take in that, when stressed and anxious, it's easy to forget.

He didn't reply, so I said, 'I'm a foster carer and I live here with my family. We are going to look after you, as your mummy can't at present.'

I would have expected a child of his age to understand the concept phrased this way. Miss Jordan, his teacher, had said Oskar had a good grasp of English and his learning was above average. But Oskar looked at me blankly and then asked, 'Does Mummy look after me?'

'Yes, I think so. Usually.' That was the impression I'd been given and what his social worker and teacher believed. But Oskar was looking bewildered, and given we knew so little about him, I thought I should try to clarify this. 'Did your mummy look after you before she went away?' I asked.

'Looked after?' he repeated questioningly.

'Yes, made your meals, washed your clothes, played with you.'

'No. Maybe. Sometimes,' he said, confused.

'Who else looked after you?' I asked.

He shrugged. 'I don't know all their names.'

'The uncles who took you to school?'

'Sometimes.'

The set-up at Oskar's home seemed even more complex than his social worker or school had realized. Most children who come into care have a bond with and are loyal to their main care-giver, usually a parent or relative, even if they've been neglected or abused. They often try to portray them in a more positive light than they deserve out of loyalty, but not so

15

with Oskar. He seemed to be struggling with the idea of being looked after at all.

'When Mummy is at home, does she make your meals and spend time with you?' I asked lightly, picking up a toy and approaching the matter from a different angle.

'She works,' he said, watching me.

'OK, but when she doesn't work, is she the one who takes care of you?'

He shrugged and began to look anxious, so again I let the subject drop. Once he was feeling more at ease, hopefully he'd begin to talk.

'Don't worry,' I said. 'Let's go and see how the casserole is doing.' I offered him my hand and we went into the kitchen, where Oskar waited a safe distance from the hot oven as I opened the door and gave the casserole a stir.

'Hmm, that smells nice,' he said.

'Good. Another fifteen minutes and it will be ready to eat. What would you like to drink with your meal?'

'Water, please.'

I poured a tumbler of water and set it at his place on the table. We tend to keep the same places at the meal table, as many families do. I showed Oskar his place. I was expecting Adrian and Lucy to arrive home at any moment and I'd just begun telling him a little bit about them when I heard Lucy let herself in the front door. 'Hi, Mum!' she shouted, making Oskar start.

'Quietly, Lucy,' I called. She bounced into the kitchen.

'Hi, Oskar,' she cried, delighted to see him. She was a qualified nursery assistant and I knew that sometimes she'd been asked to quell her exuberance at work, but I was pleased she was so outgoing and happy. It had been very different when she'd first come to me as a foster child, withdrawn and with

an eating disorder. (I tell Lucy's story in *Will You Love Me?*)
She'd done amazingly well and was now a permanent
member of my family. I'd adopted her and loved her as much
as I did my birth children – Adrian and Paula.

Having said a few words to Oskar, Lucy went upstairs to
change out of her work clothes. Five minutes later Adrian
arrived home, making a slightly more reserved entrance. He
came in, said hello to Oskar, kissed my cheek, asked if I'd had
a good day and then went upstairs to change. I gave him and
Lucy a few minutes and then called everyone to dinner. I
dished up and we settled around the table to eat.

I always anticipate that our new arrival may feel uncomfortable for the first few days, surrounded by new people and
customs, especially at the meal table when we are all in close
proximity and the noise level rises as we talk about our day.
Lucy entertained us with a funny story about a child at nursery, and Adrian said a little about his day at work as a trainee
accountant. Paula talked of her day at college, and I of fostering and the part-time clerical work I did mainly from home.

As we chatted and ate, I watched Oskar but he didn't seem
to mind all the talking or being surrounded by new people.
He ate well and had seconds, and a pudding. It was later, after
dinner, when I began his bedtime routine, that his anxiety set
in again. I'd read him a story in the living room and at seven
o'clock I said it was time for bed.

'Do I have to sleep upstairs?' he asked.

'Yes, love, that's where the beds are.'

'Can I sleep on the floor downstairs?'

'No, that would be very uncomfortable,' I said. 'Do you
sleep in a bed at your home?' I'd fostered children before
who'd had to sleep on the sofa or a mattress on the floor
because there wasn't money for a bed.

He didn't reply but came with me to the bathroom, where I'd set out a fresh towel, toothbrush, soap, sponge, clean pyjamas and so forth from my spares.

'I don't want a bath,' he said as soon as we went in.

'Would you like a shower instead?' I asked.

'No.' He began to look worried again.

'OK, just have a good wash tonight. I expect you're tired. You can have a bath tomorrow.' I never usually insist a child has a bath or shower on their first night; I wait until they feel more comfortable with me.

I ran water for him in the washbasin and then waited while he washed his face, going carefully over his cheek where the bruise was. 'That looks sore,' I said.

He shrugged. I thought Miss Jordan had done well to get Oskar talking about how he got the mark on his face, as he was saying so little to me. But she'd had a term – four months – to gain his trust, while I'd only had a few hours. I hoped in time he'd start to trust me and open up. He washed his hands and brushed his teeth, then I handed him his pyjamas.

'Do you need help changing into your pyjamas or shall I wait outside?' I asked him, respecting his privacy.

'I want to sleep in my clothes,' he said, immediately growing anxious. 'Please let me sleep in my clothes.' His eyes filled.

An icy chill ran up my spine. I hoped I was wrong, but a child not wanting to undress can be a sign that they've been sexually abused.

CHAPTER THREE

PROTECTING OSKAR

Preoccupied with Oskar's reaction to changing into his night clothes, I picked up his pyjamas and we went round the landing to his bedroom. I certainly wouldn't be forcing him to change, but I hoped to be able to persuade him, and also to find out the reason for his reluctance to undress. There might be a perfectly innocent explanation, although as a very experienced foster carer I had my doubts.

It was still light outside and I asked Oskar if he liked to sleep with his curtains closed, open or open a little. On their first night I always ask a child this and other questions regarding how they like their bedroom. It's small details like this that help them settle in a strange room. He replied, 'I think they're closed.'

'OK.'

'Do you like to sleep with your bedroom light on or off? Or I can dim it a little if you wish.' I thought if I made his room as he was used to then he'd start to feel more secure.

He didn't reply so I showed him what I meant by switching the light on and off and then dimming it. 'On or off?' I asked again. 'Or dimmed?'

'It goes on and off a lot,' he said. 'It wakes me up.'

'You mean the light flashes?' I asked, slightly baffled. I wondered if he lived in a built-up area where car headlights caught his bedroom window, or possibly a neon shop sign flashed on and off late at night.

'They keep switching it on,' Oskar said.

'Who do?' I asked.

'The people in the house.'

'Oh. What people are they, love?'

He clammed up again. So often in fostering the child is reluctant to confide to begin with and foster carers (and social workers) have to become detectives, gently easing the information from them. We also have to be receptive if a child starts to tell us something, as what they are really trying to say may not be obvious.

'This room is your bedroom and only you sleep here,' I emphasized, hoping to make him feel safe. 'I won't come into your room and switch on the light unless you want me to. You can have your door open or closed, just as you wish. When it is time to get up for school, I will knock on your door to wake you and then you can call out, "Come in."'

'Knock on my door,' he repeated, as though he hadn't a clue what I was talking about.

'Yes, like this.' I stepped outside, drew the door to, knocked on it and said, 'It's Cathy, can I come in? Then you say, "Yes, come in."'

I demonstrated again and on the second try he called out, 'Yes, come in.'

'Great,' I said. 'Well done. Remember, it's your room. You're in charge of it. OK?'

He nodded, and at that point I think he began to accept that he was going to be safe, for his face lost some of its unease and he started looking around the room. There wasn't really much to see without his possessions: furniture, posters on the walls, and I'd put in a toy box and some soft toys. Now he was more relaxed I thought I'd ask him to change. I really needed him to change into night clothes so I could wash his school uniform, and I didn't want him to start a habit of sleeping every night in his day clothes.

'Oskar, I'm going to wait outside while you change into your pyjamas and get into bed. Then, once you are ready, you can call out "come in".' Without waiting for a refusal, I stepped outside the door, drew it to and waited. A few minutes later his little voice rang out. 'I'm in bed. You can come in.' I smiled.

Even so, I knocked on the door before I went in. 'Well done,' I said, and scooped up his day clothes. 'I'll wash these ready for school tomorrow.'

'Will you take me to school?' he asked, his little face peeping over the duvet.

'Yes, and collect you. Now I want you to try to get some sleep. You've had a very tiring day. Would you like a goodnight kiss?' I always check, otherwise it can be an uncomfortable invasion of the child's personal space and terrifying for those who have been abused.

Oskar shook his head and looked worried. 'It's fine, you don't have to have a kiss. I'll just say goodnight and see you in the morning. Call out if you need me.' I tucked him in and went to the door. 'Would you like your door left open, closed or a little open?' I asked him again.

'Closed,' he said.

'OK.'

Leaving the light on low, I came out convinced there was far more going on for Oskar than anyone knew.

* * *

Downstairs, I put his clothes in the washer-dryer and then checked his school's website for its start and finish times. After that, I set about writing up my log notes while I had the chance. All foster carers in the UK are required to keep a daily record of the child or children they are looking after. This includes appointments, the child's health and well-being, education, significant events and any disclosures the child may make about their past. As well as charting the child's progress, it can act as an aide-mémoire. When the child leaves, this record is placed on file at the social services. Some carers type these, but I'm not alone in preferring to keep a written record and then emailing a résumé as part of my monthly report to the child's social worker and my supervising social worker.

As I wrote, I included collecting Oskar from school, that he'd eaten a good meal, how he appeared to be coping with being in care and his comments where appropriate. The account has to be objective, so I didn't include that I thought there was far more going on in Oskar's life than anyone knew about. This was conjecture at present and time would tell if I was right or not. Once I'd completed my notes for the day, I stored the folder in a locked drawer in the front room with other important paperwork.

I went upstairs and quietly checked on Oskar. He was fast asleep. I then spent some time talking to Adrian, Paula and Lucy, who thought Oskar was a lovely boy but looked very troubled – 'as though he has the weight of the world on his shoulders', Paula said. This wasn't altogether surprising considering he'd just come into care, regardless of whatever else might have happened in his past. I said I hoped that in time he would start to relax and look a bit happier, as other children we'd fostered had. Generally, children have amazing resilience and adapt to change – in my opinion, they are all little heroes.

Aware that Oskar would probably have an unsettled first night, I went to bed shortly after ten o'clock. I never sleep well when there is a new child in the house. I'm half listening out in case they wake frightened, not knowing where they are and in need of reassurance. I checked on Oskar around 2.00 a.m., and when I woke at 6.00 he was still asleep. Indeed, he slept through until 7.00, when I gently woke him to get ready for school.

'Where am I?' he asked, sitting bolt upright in bed.

'You're staying with me, Cathy,' I said quietly.

'Oh yes, I remember.' He rubbed his eyes.

I now expected him to ask me when he would see his mummy, as most children would. He'd hardly mentioned her the evening before and he didn't now. He simply got out of bed, used the toilet, and then I left him to change into his school uniform that I'd laundered the night before. I'd buy another school uniform today, as we couldn't get by on one and I didn't know if or when his clothes would be sent from home. Sometimes parents send their child's belongings once they are less upset and angry about their child going into care, others don't, in which case I replace the lot.

I waited on the landing while Oskar dressed and then took him downstairs for breakfast, talking to him and reassuring him. Although he wasn't saying much, he still looked anxious. Adrian and Lucy were already at the table having their breakfasts and said hi to Oskar. He looked at them warily. Paula didn't have to leave as early as they did and would come down shortly. On a weekday my family usually fix their own breakfasts and then at the weekend, when there is more time, I often make a cooked breakfast.

At dinner the evening before, Oskar had sat next to Adrian where I'd laid his place, but this morning he seemed to purposely go around him to the other side of the table. He sat next to Lucy, as far away from Adrian as possible. 'I'm honoured,' Lucy said with a smile, having also noticed Oskar's decision. It was where Paula usually sat at the table, but she wouldn't mind.

'What would you like for breakfast?' I asked Oskar. 'Cereal, toast, yoghurt, fruit?'

He looked confused. 'Would you like to come and see what we have?' I suggested.

'You can choose what you want,' Lucy prompted when he didn't move.

'Within reason,' I added. I wasn't about to let him have a chocolate bar and fizzy drink for breakfast, as some children I'd fostered were used to. Foster carers are expected to provide healthy, nutritious meals for their family and the children they look after.

Oskar slid quietly from his chair and came into the kitchen, where I opened the cupboard doors and the fridge to show him the choices. He didn't seem to spot anything he might like. I opened the bread bin. 'Or toast?' I asked him.

'I have rolls, a bit like those,' he said, pointing, clearly used to something different.

I took out the bag of wholemeal rolls. 'Would you like these for now and then after school we can go to the supermarket and you can show me what you like to eat?'

He nodded.

'How many rolls?'

'One,' he said.

'What would you like in it?'

24

I showed him what we had and he chose ham and a slice of cheese as a filling, and a drink of orange juice. By the time he sat down at the table to eat, Adrian and Lucy were leaving to get ready for work. I took my coffee and sat with Oskar as he ate. It wasn't long before the smell of ham brought Sammy in, nose twitching. I gave him a stroke and then kept an eye on him, making sure he didn't jump up and steal some ham, as he tried to do sometimes.

'Do you like the cat?' Oskar asked me as he ate.

'Yes.' I smiled. 'He's like one of the family. Do you have a pet?'

'At my house …' he began, and stopped.

'Yes, love?'

But he continued eating, clearly having decided not to say any more on that topic. Then he asked, 'Can we go to school now?'

'When you've finished your breakfast. There's no rush.'

Paula appeared and said hi to us both before getting herself some breakfast. She sat next to me and we talked a little about her college as Oskar finished his roll and then drank the juice.

'Can we go to school now?' he asked again the moment he'd finished.

'Yes, but there's plenty of time. We won't be late.' Given that he'd often been late for school in the past, I guessed it was worrying him.

'Have a good day,' Paula said as Oskar and I left the table.

'And you, love,' I replied.

I took Oskar upstairs to wash his face and hands and brush his teeth, and then downstairs again we put on our jackets and shoes. He appeared to be very self-sufficient and didn't need much help from me.

'Are we going to school now?' he asked as we got into the car.

'Yes, but don't worry, you won't be late.'

He asked me again as I drove and I said, 'We're going to school, but it's a different route to the one you're used to, as I live in a different part of town.'

'I like school,' he said.

'Good, I'm pleased.'

'I like school,' he said again a minute later. 'I wish I could stay there.'

I glanced at him in the rear-view mirror. He was looking out of his side window, frowning, deep in thought as he often seemed to be.

'Why do you prefer school to home?' I asked gently. Many children like school, but preferring it to home was unusual and also worrying. I'd had children before disclose abuse while I'd been driving. I think it helps, not being able to see the person's face when saying something painful, similar to writing it down or confiding in a diary.

Oskar hadn't replied, but he was still frowning and continued to gaze out of his side window.

'Why is school better than your home?' I asked again lightly, keeping my eyes on the road ahead. 'Can you think of a reason?'

'My teacher is nice,' he offered.

'Yes. She is nice,' I agreed. Although that alone wouldn't normally be enough for a child to prefer school to home.

'Are the people in your house nice?' I asked.

He didn't reply, but as I looked again in the rear-view mirror I saw him imperceptibly shake his head and his frown deepen.

'Oskar, love, is there anything about your home life that is worrying you and you can tell me? I know you were able to

26

tell Miss Jordan some things yesterday and that was very brave of you. Is there anything else you want to say?' He didn't reply. 'If you do think of anything, you know you can tell me or Miss Jordan. We are both here to help you.'

But he changed the subject. 'There's a cat like Sammy,' he said, pointing through the window.

'Yes, he is,' I agreed.

I parked outside Oskar's school and he couldn't get out of the car fast enough, his face losing some of its angst. As soon as we entered the playground, Miss Jordan appeared. I think she must have been looking out for us. She came straight over.

'My teacher!' Oskar cried, delighted.

'How are you, Oskar?' she asked emotionally. I know teachers aren't supposed to encourage physical contact with their pupils, but she allowed him a hug.

'He's doing fine,' I told her. 'He had a good night's sleep and is eating well.'

'That's a relief. I had a sleepless night worrying about him.' I knew how she felt! 'I'm sure he's looking better already, less tired,' she said. I had thought so too – the dark rings under his eyes were fading. 'Can you come into reception?' she asked me. 'The secretary needs you to fill in a form with your contact details. There wasn't time yesterday.'

'Yes. I also need to buy Oskar another school uniform,' I said.

'You might not have to. Oskar's uncle, Mr Nowak, has just brought in a big bag of Oskar's belongings.'

'Really? That was quick.' I was surprised, but pleased Oskar was going to be reunited with some of his possessions.

We followed Miss Jordan into reception where she introduced me to the school secretary, then she waited, talking to

Oskar, while I filled in the necessary form. I asked the secretary if Oskar's school dinners had been paid for. When a child comes into care this becomes the carer's responsibility and often the bill hasn't been settled, so I pay it straight away. The secretary checked on her computer and said Oskar's school meals had been paid for until half-term, so nothing was outstanding.

Miss Jordan then went into the office and brought out a large laundry-style bag that Mr Nowak had dropped off. 'Will you be able to manage it?' she asked, setting the bag on the floor beside me.

'Yes, I should think so,' I said, testing it. 'I've got my car outside.' It was bulky rather than very heavy.

Oskar was looking at the bag. 'I'll take this home and put your things in your bedroom,' I said to him.

He didn't reply.

'Oskar's PE kit and book bag are in the classroom,' Miss Jordan said. 'I didn't bother you with them yesterday.' I nodded. 'We like the PE kit to be taken home and washed once a week, and the book bag goes home with the child every afternoon so they can read a little.' This was usual for a primary school.

'Where should I wait for Oskar at the end of school?' I asked.

'In the front playground, where you came in,' Miss Jordan replied. 'The teachers bring out their classes. In the morning the children come in from the same place.' Again, this wasn't dissimilar to other schools. 'As there is only five minutes before the start of school, Oskar can come with me for now and wait in my classroom,' Miss Jordan offered.

'Thank you.'

I said goodbye to Oskar and told him I would meet him at the end of school in the playground.

'Am I going home with you again?' he asked. I was reminded of just how confusing it is for a child to come into foster care.

'Yes, love. You will be staying with me for a while. Have a good day and I'll see you when school finishes.'

Oskar went with Miss Jordan, while I picked up the bag and left the building. I would see what clothes had been sent for Oskar before I bought a new school uniform or casual clothes. It's preferable for the child if they can wear what they are used to, as it's familiar and comforting.

With only five minutes to go before the start of school, the playground had filled with parents, carers and their children. As I made my way towards the main gate with the cumbersome laundry bag bumping against my leg, I heard a shout of, 'Cathy!'

I turned and there was Angela, another foster carer I knew from attending foster-carer training and support groups. I set down the bag and we hugged and then had a chat. She was fostering a brother and sister who attended the school and who she said should be going home to their mother before too long, which was good. It wasn't a huge coincidence that I'd bumped into a fellow foster carer. Having been fostering for over twenty-five years in the same area, I knew many foster carers and I had, at one time or another, stood in most school playgrounds in the county. It's always nice to see a familiar face.

When the klaxon sounded for the start of school, we said goodbye and I picked up the bag and continued out of the school gates. As I did, my gaze fell on a car parked on the opposite side of the road. I was sure it was the same black car with two men in it that I'd seen the afternoon before. Whether it had been there when Oskar and I had come into school I didn't know; I'd been looking in the opposite direction, towards the school. They were both looking at me. I continued to my car and, once in, I pressed the central locking system. I doubted they were parents, as they would have been in the playground seeing in their children. Perhaps one of them was Mr Nowak, who had dropped off Oskar's belongings.

I started the car and pulled away, and the black car headed off in the opposite direction. If they were there again this afternoon, I would ask Miss Jordan or the school secretary if they knew who they were. Children in care are sometimes snatched by a family member from outside their school, and foster carers are advised not to put up a struggle and risk being hurt, but to let the child go and immediately call the social services and the police. Thankfully it doesn't happen often, and it had never happened to me. But, of course, there is always a first time, so I needed to stay alert to protect Oskar.

CHAPTER FOUR

STRESSED AND TENSE

I arrived home still slightly unsettled from seeing the men waiting outside school. Had Oskar not recognized them the day before and then denied knowing them it probably wouldn't have played on my mind, but he had recognized them – I was sure of it. However, aware I was likely to have a busy day, I thought it wise to unpack Oskar's bag straight away. The first few days after a new child arrives are usually very busy and I was expecting to be spending a lot of time on the phone. I heaved the bag upstairs, along the landing and into Oskar's bedroom. It was a fine spring day outside and the sun streamed through his bedroom window. I opened it a little and then unzipped the bag and began sorting through it.

It looked to me as though whoever had packed the bag had just grabbed whatever clothes of Oskar's had come to hand. Some of them needed washing and I put those to one side, others had been washed but not ironed. There was a pair of pyjamas that looked too small for Oskar, a pair of grey school trousers, well-worn blue joggers, various socks (which I paired), some underpants, a vest, a zip-up jacket, new trainers and an old bath towel. There were also four small plastic toy cars. All in all, it was a meagre and rather sad selection, but I set about putting the clean clothes in his drawers and the toy cars on a shelf in his room. There is a great temptation as a foster carer – wanting the best for the child – to discard old possessions and replace them all with new. I would be buying Oskar plenty of new clothes (and toys), but I wouldn't be getting rid of his old things. These would be a poignant reminder of – and link to – home, and also legally they belonged to his mother.

Having put away the clean clothes and the bag they came in, I scooped up the items that needed washing and took them downstairs, where I put them in the washer-dryer with the rest of the laundry. Not a moment too soon, for as the machine began its cycle the landline rang. I answered it in the kitchen and it was Andrew, Oskar's social worker.

'Good morning. What sort of night did Oskar have?' he asked.

'Good. No tears. He slept well. Although it appears he's used to sleeping with his mother and some other women. I don't know who they are. He gave me some names but said they weren't his sisters, cousins or friends.'

'How many women?'

'He mentioned three. I wrote their names in my log; shall I fetch it?'

'Not now. I'll know more when I've spoken to his mother, but from what Mr Nowak told me yesterday it seems they live in a multiple-occupancy house and share childcare.'

'That would make sense,' I said. 'Although Oskar was very vague about them. He didn't say much. I got the feeling they weren't close. But he had a good dinner and breakfast,' I continued. 'And is now in school.'

'Yes, I've just spoken to the Head. I understand Mr Nowak brought in some of Oskar's belongings.' Schools and social services work closely together in matters of child protection.

'Yes, I've unpacked them,' I said. 'There are some clothes and a few toy cars, but I'll need to buy more and also another school uniform.'

'OK.' I assumed Andrew was making some notes. 'Any behaviour issues?' he asked.

'Not so far, although it's early days. Oskar is very quiet and withdrawn at present, but not upset. He didn't want a bath or shower last night, and I didn't insist.' This point wasn't just about hygiene; it meant I hadn't had a chance to check Oskar to see if he had any injuries apart from the bruise on his cheek.

'I'm going to arrange a medical for him, hopefully for later today,' Andrew said. It's usual for a child to have a medical when they first come into care, but it can sometimes take a few days to organize. 'Oskar's mother is still abroad, but I've left a message on her voicemail to phone me. Has Oskar said any more about how he got the bruise on his cheek?'

'No.'

'Are there any other injuries you can see?'

'No. But I haven't seen him undressed. He wanted to sleep in his clothes to begin with. I persuaded him to change, but I had to wait outside his bedroom door while he did so.'

'I see. I'll sort out a medical. That should pick up anything else. You're keeping a note of all this?'

'Yes.'

'Thanks. I'll be in touch about the medical and also I'll need to visit Oskar and you later in the week.' When a child is placed in care the social worker is duty-bound to visit the child within the first week and then at least every six weeks for the first year.

We said goodbye, and I thought while I had the phone in my hand I should phone my supervising social worker, Edith, and update her. My call went through to her voicemail, so I left a message saying that Oskar had had a good night, was now in school and I'd updated his social worker. If she needed to know more, she'd phone me.

Now I'd gone through Oskar's bag of belongings from home I had a better idea of what I needed to buy for him, so I made a list, downed a quick coffee and then drove into town. I'd just parked when my mobile rang. It was Andrew again. 'I've arranged for Oskar to have a medical at the Health Centre this afternoon at two-thirty,' he said. 'I'm emailing the form to the clinic now. I'll inform his school that you will be collecting Oskar early today. How much time will you need?'

'Half an hour to be on the safe side, so I'll have to collect him at two o'clock.' I'd taken children to the Health Centre before, so I knew where it was.

'I'll tell them,' Andrew said.

'Any news from Oskar's mother yet?' I asked.

'No.'

Having said goodbye, I headed for the shops, list in hand, where I quickly set about buying Oskar the items he needed. I could tell by looking at the clothes if they would fit him; I'm a reasonable judge after years of looking after children, as most parents and carers are. I bought him two sets of pyjamas patterned with pictures of dinosaurs, a dressing gown, slippers, casual clothes, socks, underwear and grey school trousers. The T-shirts and jerseys showing the school's emblem could only be bought from his school. I was hoping I'd have time to buy those later when I collected Oskar for his medical. Andrew had arranged the medical very quickly and I assumed it was because Oskar had suffered at least one suspected non-accidental injury – the bruise to his face – and might have more, so it was prudent to have him examined as soon as possible. Had he had more serious injuries, he would have been taken to hospital to be treated and examined.

On the way out of the shopping centre I stopped off at the department store where I knew they had a good selection of cute, cuddly soft toys. I think all children need at least one cuddly toy they can hold close, take to bed if they wish and draw comfort from. Oskar might already have one at home, but it hadn't been packed. After some deliberation – I could have bought the lot – I chose a traditional teddy bear with very soft brown fur. When my children were young and I had to re-equip a child we were fostering with virtually everything, I used to buy them a little gift to redress the balance, otherwise it could have seemed like favouritism. They didn't expect it, and appreciated that they had plenty of clothes and belongings while the fostered child often had very little, but I felt better for doing it. Now they were older they often bought the child small gifts too, which was nice of them. It doesn't take much to bring a smile to a child's face. But of course, the best gift of all is to be shown kindness, attention and respect.

Once home, I made a sandwich lunch, which I ate as I put together a pasta bake for dinner later, then it was time to set off to Oskar's school. I arrived outside at 1.45 p.m., buzzed the security-locked outer gate and a few seconds later it released. I crossed the empty playground and buzzed the entry system on the main door.

'You're early,' the school secretary said a little curtly as I entered. 'I was told to expect you at two o'clock.' She was in the open-plan office to the right and was clearly very busy.

'I was hoping I could buy Oskar some school T-shirts and jerseys,' I said. 'He only has one with him.'

'We sell them at the end of school,' she said, concentrating on her computer screen.

'Shall I wait until tomorrow afternoon?' I asked. 'I won't be returning to school today.'

There was a moment's silence when I thought I might have heard a tut, and then she stood and asked, 'What size and how many?'

'Two of each, please. Aged six.'

She disappeared out the back of the office while I waited in reception. A few minutes later she reappeared with the garments in plastic bags. I thanked her and paid. 'You can go up and collect him now if you like,' she said. 'It's nearly two o'clock. Sign in the Visitors' Book first.'

I thanked her again, signed the book and made my way to Oskar's classroom, feeling like a chastised child. Much has changed since I was at school, but it doesn't take much for me to be transported back to my own school days. The sounds, smells, classrooms, assembly hall, terse comments – they all form poignant reminders, good and bad.

I looked through the glass panel in the door of Oskar's classroom and saw Miss Jordan moving between the tables as the children worked. She saw me and nodded, then brought Oskar to me. 'Thank you,' I said.

'See you tomorrow,' she smiled, and returned to her class.

'Where are we going?' Oskar asked, worried, as we went along the corridor.

I was sure Miss Jordan would have told him, but I explained. 'To the Health Centre so a doctor can check you over and make sure you are healthy. There is nothing for you to worry about.'

We entered reception and I signed out of the Visitors' Book as the school secretary watched from the office, then I pressed the button to release the main door.

'Have you ever seen a doctor before?' I asked Oskar as we crossed the playground.

'Yes, I had a cough, but I'm not ill now.'

'I know. This is to make sure you stay well. The doctor will weigh and measure you, listen to your chest, check your eyes and ears and probably feel your tummy. It's nothing for you to worry about,' I said again, for Oskar was still looking very serious. 'I bought you some new clothes today,' I said, changing the subject. 'And a little present.'

Most children would have asked what the present was, but Oskar didn't. He got silently into the car and remained quiet as I drove. 'Are you all right?' I asked him after a while.

'Yes,' he said, but in a way that didn't reassure me at all.

'You know you can tell me if there is something worrying you,' I said, as I had said previously, and would say again.

'Yes,' he said quietly.

'Did you have a good morning at school?'

He didn't reply but gazed out of his side window, deep in thought.

'What's your favourite subject?' I asked, trying to engage him.

'Science,' he said in a deadpan voice.

I continued talking to him and then I fed a CD of popular children's songs into the player. Oskar was quiet all the way to the Health Centre and then held my hand as we crossed the car park. I gave his name to the receptionist and said we were there for his medical. She told us to take a seat in the waiting area. The centre ran various clinics for children and adults, including immunizations, well-woman check-ups, blood tests and dentistry. Some of the children were playing with the toys provided, but Oskar just wanted to sit beside me. I picked up one of the children's story books, but he was too preoccupied to take an interest. I tried talking to him, but he was locked in thought. I reassured him again that the medical was nothing to worry about. Another few minutes passed and then Oskar's name flashed on the digital display screen together with a recorded voice giving his name and telling us to go to Consulting Room 2. He started and looked at me, petrified. 'It's OK,' I said. 'It's telling us it's our turn.'

I took his hand and we went down a short corridor until we came to a door marked Consulting Room 2.

I knocked and a female voice called, 'Come in.'

As we entered, a young woman doctor seated at a desk swivelled her chair round to greet us. 'Hello, I'm Doctor Yazdi, and you must be Oskar.' She smiled pleasantly.

'Yes,' I replied on Oskar's behalf, as he'd said nothing.

'And you're Cathy Glass, his foster carer,' she said, glancing at her computer screen.

'That's right.'

'Take a seat, please.'

We sat in the two chairs at right angles to her desk. She was very nice, but Oskar was frowning harder than ever now and his legs were jumping up and down agitatedly. 'There's nothing to worry about,' I told him.

The doctor smiled. 'And you're six?' she said to him.

He managed a small nod.

'When did he come to you?' she asked me.

'Yesterday.'

'Does he have bruises anywhere else apart from his cheek?' she asked, glancing up. I assumed it was mentioned in the online form Andrew had sent for her to complete.

'Not as far as I know, but I haven't seen him undressed.'

'OK. Good boy. Let's start by having a look in your ears,' she said to Oskar with a smile. 'Can you hear all right?'

He gave a small nod. She took an otoscope from a drawer in her desk and looked in both of Oskar's ears. He didn't seem to mind, although I know it can feel a bit unpleasant. 'They're fine,' she said, then typed in the result. She returned the otoscope to the drawer and took a wooden tongue depressor from a sealed packet and then asked Oskar to open his mouth so she could examine his mouth and throat. He did as she asked.

'That's all fine,' she said, throwing the depressor in the bin. 'And his teeth are in good condition.' I threw Oskar a reassuring smile.

She then checked his eyes. 'Do you wear glasses?' she asked. Oskar shook his head.

'Can you read the letters on that chart?' She pointed to the Snellen eye chart on the wall.

Oskar stared at her.

'Does he know his letters?' she asked me.

'Yes,' I said. 'He's learning to read.'

'Read the top line for me, please,' she told him.

Finally, he did. Slowly, in a small, plaintive voice, he began reading from the top, enough to confirm he could see all right.

'Good boy,' Dr Yazdi said with another cheerful smile. 'His immunization programme is up to date,' she said to me, glancing at the screen.

'Is it? I didn't know.'

'According to our records it is, although the immunizations weren't done in this clinic. Now, let's weigh and measure you,' she said to Oskar. 'Can you stand on these scales for me?'

He didn't move, so I took his hand and helped him onto the scales by the doctor's desk. 'His weight is at the lower end of average,' she said. 'Does he have a good appetite?'

'From what I've seen, yes, but I understand he used to sometimes arrive at school hungry, which was one of the concerns.'

'He could do with putting on a few pounds,' she said, making a note. 'Let's see how tall you are,' she said to Oskar, and drew him to the height bar. 'Again, it's the lower end of average,' she said. 'But nothing to worry about. He'll probably have a growth spurt.'

I threw Oskar another reassuring smile and he looked back at me, expressionless.

'Now I'd like you to come and sit on the couch so I can listen to your chest,' Dr Yazdi said.

Oskar didn't move, so I took his hand and led him to the couch.

'Can you climb up onto it?' she asked, pulling out a step stool from beneath.

Oskar shook his head.

'I'm sure you can, a big boy like you,' Dr Yazdi encouraged.

It wasn't high and could be managed by the average two-year-old, but Oskar stood still, head down, staring at the floor.

'Up you get,' she said, 'and sit on the couch for me.'

I touched his shoulder and reluctantly Oskar did as she asked. Her stethoscope was already looped around her neck. As she went to raise Oskar's jersey at the front so she could listen to his chest he grabbed it and pulled it back down again.

'What's the matter?' she asked, concerned.

He shook his head and clutched his jersey so tightly to him his knuckles were white.

'There's nothing to worry about,' I reassured him.

'I just want to listen to your chest, Oskar,' Dr Yazdi said. 'Look, like this.' She slipped the chestpiece into the front of her blouse and put in the earpieces. 'I can hear my heart beating. Would you like a listen?'

A trained paediatrician, she was so patient. She allowed him a listen and then gradually Oskar released his jersey and let her lift it up so she could listen to his chest and then his back. This also gave her the opportunity to check his skin for any more bruising or suspicious marks. I couldn't see any.

'His heart and lungs are fine,' she said to me. Then to Oskar, 'Good boy. Now I want you to lie down so I can feel your tummy. And I'll have a look at your arms and legs too. Have you been to the toilet today?'

Oskar didn't reply, so I said, 'Yes, he went this morning.'

'Good, and he takes care of his own hygiene?'

'Yes,' I confirmed.

'Lie flat on your back then,' she told Oskar, who hadn't moved. 'It's not going to hurt.' He still didn't move.

'Lie down, love,' I said. 'It's part of the medical. I'll hold your hand if you like.'

He gave me his hand and gradually I eased him down, but I could feel how tense he was.

'He's very anxious,' Dr Yazdi commented. 'Is he always like this?'

'He's been very quiet since he arrived, but he hasn't been this tense.'

'Don't you like doctors?' she asked him with a smile.

Oskar stared back, petrified.

'It won't take long,' she said. 'Let's have a look at your arms and legs first then.' She began by easing up his trouser legs as far as they would go to the knees and examining his legs.

'They're fine,' she said. Then she looked at his arms and moved up his jersey. With a flat hand she began lightly pressing his stomach. Oskar shut his eyes, held his breath and grimaced.

'I'm not hurting you, am I?' the doctor asked, pausing, concerned.

He didn't reply but kept his eyes screwed tightly shut. She glanced at me and then moved her hand to his lower abdomen. Oskar went rigid. He was so still and tense that for a moment I thought he was going to fit.

'OK, that's enough,' the doctor said. 'You can get off the couch.' I helped him down. 'From what I can see he appears healthy, but he's very anxious. I'll send my report to his social worker. He may want a follow-up medical in a few months when Oskar is more relaxed.'

I thanked her and helped Oskar into his jacket, then I took his hand as we left the consulting room. I wasn't reassured by hearing the doctor pronounce Oskar healthy, not at all. The only other child I'd seen so stressed at having a medical and who hadn't wanted to remove their clothes had been sexually abused. Alarm bells were ringing again, although of course it was still only a suspicion. There was no proof, and I sincerely hoped I was wrong.

CHAPTER FIVE

YOU KNOW THOSE MEN?

Oskar was just as quiet in the car on the way home from the Health Centre as he had been on the way there. I asked him a couple of times if he was all right, without much response, and then I said I was going to stop off at the super-market so he could choose some food he liked. He didn't reply but I went anyway, as I needed to top up on general food items like bread, milk, fruit and so forth.

'Would you like to push the trolley?' I asked Oskar. Most children love being in charge of a supermarket trolley, some-times to the detriment of other shoppers! Oskar shook his head, but he was content to walk beside me as we went up and down the aisles.

'Tell me if you see anything you fancy,' I said. It's not an invitation I would offer to some children, as we would end up with a trolley full of crisps, sweets, biscuits and Pot Noodles. Oskar didn't make any suggestions at all.

The supermarket, like many, had plenty of counters displaying food from other countries and I pointed these out to Oskar and lingered by them, hoping he would spot some-thing he liked, but he didn't. He wasn't interested and remained thoughtful. When we got to the bread counter, I asked him if he could see any of the rolls he had for breakfast at home. Without any enthusiasm, he took a bag of sourdough bread rolls with seeds on and passed them to me. 'Good. What would you like to go in them?'

He shrugged. 'Don't mind.'

I thought that once his social worker had spoken to his mother, I'd have a better idea of Oskar's likes and dislikes. All I knew at present was what Oskar's uncle had told Andrew: that Oskar didn't have any food allergies or special dietary requirements. But all children have food preferences, which I try to accommodate within reason. For now, however, I bought the rolls and some more ham and cheese filling, as well as the other items we needed. Oskar remained quiet and pensive as we completed the shop, and afterwards, when we were in the car going home, I asked him if there was anything wrong, but he shook his head. Then, as I drove, he suddenly asked, 'Will I have to have another medical?'

'Possibly in the future. Most children do, but it's nothing to worry about.'

'I don't like taking off my clothes,' he said.

'I know.' I glanced at him in the rear-view mirror. 'Why?'

Silence. He was staring out of his window and frowning.

'Is there any reason you don't like undressing?' I asked him. 'We all have to undress sometimes, to shower, go swimming or when we see a doctor.'

There was a long silence and then he said again, 'I don't like taking off my clothes.'

'I know, you said. Is there a reason?' There was no reply and so the matter was dropped.

Oskar and I were the only ones in when we arrived home, apart from Sammy, who, hearing us, had shot in through the cat flap in the kitchen, startling Oskar. I was unpacking the shopping and Oskar had been standing to one side, watching me. I noticed he didn't let me far out of his sight. Sammy began meowing loudly for his dinner. 'Would you like to feed him?' I asked Oskar.

He nodded.

I broke off from unpacking the groceries, took the bag of dry cat food from the cupboard and gave the scoop to Oskar. 'Just one scoop,' I said. 'Place it in his food bowl.'

Oskar fed Sammy and then watched him eat, while I finished unpacking the shopping.

'I bought you some new clothes, and there's a present for you on your bed,' I said to Oskar.

I was expecting some form of positive reaction, but to my astonishment he said, 'I don't want it.'

'But you haven't seen what it is yet,' I said, smiling.

He looked at me, wide-eyed and wary, as he often was.

'Do you want to go up and see what it is?'

He shook his head.

'OK, shall I bring it down?' Some children don't like going upstairs by themselves, and the house was still strange to him.

He didn't reply, so I went upstairs and brought down the teddy bear, which was still in the store bag. 'I hope you like it,' I said, handing it to him.

I might have been giving him hot coals for all the trepidation he showed in opening the bag. He gingerly parted the top, peered inside and looked at me.

'It won't bite. It's a cuddly teddy bear,' I said, stating the obvious. 'With lovely soft fur. We could sit him at your place at the table,' I suggested.

He handed me the bag, so I assumed he was in agreement, and I sat the bear in the chair next to Adrian's. He watched me warily but didn't say anything. 'You'll have to think of a name for him,' I suggested.

'Luka,' he said.

'That's a nice name.'

'It's my brother's.'

'Brother?' I asked, astonished. There had been no mention of a brother.

'Where does he live?' I wondered if Andrew knew of the existence of Oskar's brother, which could raise further child-protection issues.

Oskar just looked at me.

'Does your brother live with you?' I asked.

He shook his head.

'Where is he?'

'With my aunt.'

'Where?'

He shrugged.

'How old is Luka? Do you know?'

'Twelve.'

'Do you have any other brothers or sisters?'

He shook his head again.

'OK, just sit at the table for a minute and do a puzzle,' I said. 'I have to make a phone call. I won't be long. I'll be in the hall.' I took some puzzles from the toy cupboard and placed them on the table. I needed to tell Oskar's social worker what he'd said, for I felt sure Andrew would have told me if he was aware Oskar had a brother. It was important he knew as soon as possible, as it's generally felt that if one child in a family is at risk of harm then other siblings could be too, so normally it's investigated as a matter of urgency.

Andrew answered straight away. 'It's Cathy Glass, Oskar's carer.'

'Hello, I was going to phone you to arrange to see you tomorrow. Is everything all right?'

'Yes, Oskar had his medical. But I thought you should know, he's just told me he has a brother, Luka, aged twelve, apparently living with an aunt, I'm not sure where.'

'Yes, I've only just found out. I managed to speak to his mother this afternoon and she is with Luka now in —' He named the country they originally came from. 'Sorry, I'm in a hurry now, I've got to place a child with carers. Can I visit you and Oskar tomorrow after school? I'll explain then.'

'Yes, we'll be home by four o'clock.'

'Thank you.'

He said a quick goodbye and I returned to the kitchen-diner to find Oskar at the table doing the puzzle, but he had moved seats, so he was now sitting next to where Lucy sat at meal times, rather than Adrian. I didn't say anything; it didn't matter. I praised him for doing the puzzle nicely, then set about making dinner for when everyone came home. I could see Oskar seated at the table from where I worked in the kitchen, and every so often he glanced at me, then he asked in a small voice, 'Can I sit here?'

'Yes, if you want to. Don't you want to sit next to Adrian?' Most boys we fostered thought it was a huge privilege to sit next to Adrian and spend time with him. Often, they bonded with him first. Adrian was tall like his father, but gentle, sensitive, patient and a good role model for boys. His long-term girlfriend Kirsty was lovely too and worked as a primary school teacher.

Oskar hadn't replied, so I continued to prepare dinner and then laid the table. Paula was in first and I explained to her that Oskar would prefer to sit in her place next to Lucy, and of course she didn't mind and was happy to sit anywhere. We

47

all had dinner together shortly after six o'clock and Oskar enjoyed the spaghetti bolognaise, although I noticed him occasionally stealing glances at Adrian as we ate. Once we'd finished, I listened to Oskar read his school book – his teacher expected him to read each evening – while Adrian, Lucy and Paula did their own thing. After he'd read, I asked him if he wanted to play a board game, but he didn't, so I read him some stories and then began his bath and bedtime routine.

Oskar was still very quiet, but I hoped that as the days passed and he got to know us better he would become more confident and assertive. Upstairs, I ran his bath and told him that I would wait outside the door while he washed and to call me if he needed any help. Most children his age aren't self-conscious about being naked and I often help them in the bath by washing their necks and backs, which tend to get forgotten. Oskar clearly needed his privacy for whatever reason – and that might simply have been from living in a multiple-occupancy house where, doubtless, it was at a premium.

Oskar pushed the bathroom door right to before he undressed. I heard the water stir as he climbed into the bath and began washing himself.

'Are you OK?' I asked after a couple of minutes.

'Yes, don't come in,' was his reply.

'I won't.'

I heard more water splash and, a few minutes later, the sound of him getting out. When he opened the door, he was in his new dinosaur pyjamas.

'Very smart,' I said. I waited while he brushed his teeth and then we went round the landing to his bedroom. 'Do you want Luka, your teddy bear?' I asked him. He'd left it downstairs.

'Yes,' he said. While he used the toilet, I went downstairs and fetched the bear, and he snuggled into bed with it beside him on the pillow.

I said goodnight and came out.

Who knew what memories that bear brought back now it was named after his brother? There was so much I didn't know about Oskar and his family situation. I had many questions that needed answering, and I hoped to learn more the following afternoon when Andrew visited. So often in fostering, a child arrives and then their backstory gradually follows, unfolding piecemeal over weeks and months, until eventually a clearer picture emerges, and it's often heart-breaking. Many of these children have had to cope with so much before they come into care.

Oskar slept well, and in the morning, when I woke him and told him it was time to get ready for school, I thought he seemed marginally more relaxed. I laid out his clean school clothes and waited outside his bedroom door while he dressed, then we went downstairs together. He sat in the place he had chosen next to Lucy and wanted one of the sourdough rolls we'd bought, with a cheese and ham filling and a glass of juice. Afterwards, he went up to the bathroom by himself to wash his face and clean his teeth.

I was feeling quite optimistic as I drove to Oskar's school. The sun was out, Oskar seemed slightly more relaxed, we were establishing a routine and Oskar's social worker was vising us this afternoon with the background information that should help me better meet Oskar's needs. While not talkative in the car, Oskar did tell me he liked going to school, liked his teacher and science lessons. 'Excellent,' I said.

I parked where there was a space a little way from the school and opened Oskar's car door, which was child-locked. He slipped his hand into mine and we walked along the pavement towards the school gates. Suddenly I felt his hand grip mine and I followed his gaze. The black car was pulling up and parking on the opposite side of the road. There was no mistake. It was the same car with the two men in the front.

'You know those men, don't you?' I asked Oskar. He had quickened his pace towards the school gates, pulling me along, but didn't reply. 'Who are they? Can you tell me? You're obviously worried.'

He continued, without answering, into the playground where others were waiting for the start of school. Oskar kept his back to the road and faced the school, while I turned to look at the car. It was too far away to clearly make out the features of the men, but I could see they were both staring in our direction.

'Is it nearly time to go in?' Oskar asked me anxiously.

I glanced at my watch. 'Just a few minutes more. Do you ever see that car parked outside the school during playtime?' I asked him. At morning break and after lunch the children played out here in the playground.

He didn't reply, but his face was pinched and white.

I hesitated and then, taking Oskar's hand, I said, 'We'll go into school now. I want to try to speak to your teacher.' He didn't ask why.

I took him to the main door, where I pressed the buzzer and waited to be admitted. I thought Miss Jordan might know who the men were, and if she didn't, I would alert her to my concerns.

The door released and we went in. A smartly dressed middle-aged woman was in reception, apparently having been talking to the secretary. She smiled at Oskar. 'Can I help you?' she asked me.

'I was hoping to see Miss Jordan,' I said. 'I'm Cathy Glass, Oskar's foster carer.'

'Pleased to meet you,' she said, offering her hand for shaking. 'I'm Elaine Summer, the Head Teacher here. We didn't have a chance to meet when you collected Oskar on Tuesday. How is he?'

'Quiet, but gradually settling in,' I said.

'Miss Jordan is with a parent right now. Can I help you?'

I glanced at Oskar, wondering if I should say what I had to in front of him, but decided it might actually help to reassure him. 'There's a black car parked opposite the school,' I said. 'It was there on Tuesday and yesterday morning. There are two men in it, and they seem to be watching us. Oskar appears worried by their presence and I was wondering if Miss Jordan perhaps knew who they were.'

'Let me take a look,' the Head said decisively, and she crossed to the window that looked out over the playground. 'Yes, I can see the car you mean.'

'I've seen it there this week too,' the school secretary said. Her office overlooked the playground and road.

'It might be nothing, but as a foster carer I can't be too careful,' I said.

'No, quite,' the Head agreed. 'As a school we have to be vigilant. I'll go and talk to them and see what they want.'

I felt Oskar's hand tighten in mine and I wondered if it was wise for the Head to approach the men alone, but she was already out of the door and crossing the playground. The secretary was watching her progress too as Elaine Summer went through the main gate, crossed the road, then went up to the car and tapped on the driver's window. It lowered and as we watched we saw her talking to the men for some minutes. Then she turned and headed back, and the car pulled away. The school secretary returned to her work and the Head came in. She wasn't at all flustered.

'They're saying they are family friends and know Oskar,' she said. Then to him, 'Do you know those men?'

He gave a small nod.

'Do they live in the same house as you?'

Another small nod.

'They were just making sure you were all right,' she told him, then addressing me, 'I've asked them not to wait outside the school, as it could be unsettling for Oskar. I've had to deal with similar situations with other children in care and those whose parents are divorcing. They wait outside, hoping to see their child or talk to them. That should be an end to it now, but if you do see them again, let me know.' She threw Oskar a reassuring smile, but he still looked worried.

The klaxon sounded for the start of school and the Head told Oskar, 'There's no need for you to return to the playground, you can go straight up to your classroom.'

I said goodbye to him and that I would meet him in the playground at the end of school and wished him a good day. He went off to his classroom and I let myself out of the building. I was not wholly reassured by the Head's words, no more than Oskar appeared to have been. If the two men were simply family friends wanting to make sure he was all right, why had he been so scared? It didn't make sense.

CHAPTER SIX

WARY

The rest of the day flew by with housework, my part-time clerical work and then preparing dinner for later, which I tried to do well in advance if there was a social worker visiting us after school. They often stayed for a number of hours, especially when a child was first placed, as there was always a lot to get through. I made a casserole, so it just needed popping in the oven half an hour before we wanted to eat. I messaged our Glass WhatsApp group to remind Adrian, Paula and Lucy that Oskar's social worker was likely to still be here when they arrived home. Although they were used to finding strangers in our living room, I liked to forewarn them when possible, out of courtesy, really – it was their home, after all. Also, it minimized the chance of Lucy embarrassing herself with expletives if she returned home from a trying day at work. She loved working with the children at the nursery, but she didn't always see eye to eye with the management and tended to let off steam when she first arrived home.

That afternoon as I drove to Oskar's school, it crossed my mind that the men in the black car could be there again despite the Head Teacher speaking to them. But as I parked in my usual place a little way from the school and made my way towards the main gate there was no sign of them.

Hopefully that was the end of it, although I was still puzzled and unsettled by their interest in Oskar.

The playground slowly filled with parents and carers waiting to meet their children from school. Miss Jordan had told me that Oskar had one good friend in school, and once he was more settled with us I would ask him if he would like to invite his friend home on a play date and to stay for tea. But for now, he was still adjusting to his new life with us.

The klaxon sounded from inside, signalling the end of school, and the classes began to exit the building with their form teachers. I saw Oskar straight away, standing beside Miss Jordan, and they appeared to be looking for me in the sea of faces. I gave a little wave. Miss Jordan spotted me, said something to Oskar and they came over.

'Hello,' she said with a smile. 'Elaine told me about the car and she asked me to check everything is OK.' She looked past me to the road outside. Oskar was looking too.

'It's not here,' I confirmed. 'Thank you for your help and thanks to the Head too.'

'You're welcome. I'm sure it's dealt with, but let us know straight away if you are worried at all. I've told Oskar that he is safe in school and he must tell me if he sees the car again.'

'Thank you,' I said again. She was so caring and pleasant, as was the Head.

We said goodbye and Oskar slipped his hand into mine as we left the playground. Despite my assurance that the car wasn't there, I saw him looking up and down the road as we walked. 'It's not here,' I told him. 'I've checked.'

He didn't reply, but again I wondered why he was so worried if they were really friends of the family watching out for him. I would mention it to his social worker.

'Andrew is coming to see us after school today,' I told him as I opened the rear car door for him to get in. Oskar accepted this as he accepted most things – resolutely and in silence. 'He will want to spend some time talking to you to make sure you're all right,' I continued as I started the car and pulled away. 'Then you will probably be able to go off and play while he talks to me.' This was the usual format of these visits, although so far Oskar hadn't really shown much interest in 'playing'. He'd done a jigsaw while I'd been talking on the telephone, but that was all. 'Do you watch television at home?' I asked him as I drove.

'Sometimes,' he said.

'If you tell me what your favourite programmes are, I can stream them so you can watch them on the television or my tablet.' He didn't reply, so I asked, 'What do you usually do in the evenings and at weekends?'

He thought for a moment and then said, 'Get in my sleeping bag.'

I glanced at him in the rear-view mirror. 'You mean like a camping sleeping bag?'

Silence and then, 'I think so.'

'Do you sleep in the sleeping bag at night or just use it during the day?' Perhaps it was a game he played?

Another pause and then he said, 'Both. I sleep in it.'

'So you don't sleep under a duvet like you do at my house?' I asked.

I saw him shake his head and start to look worried. However, before I let the matter drop, I had one last question.

'Oskar, do you sleep in a bed at your house?'

'No. On the floor with the others.'

'What others?'

But he'd withdrawn into his shell again and I made a mental note to mention this to his social worker too.

Once home, I fixed Oskar a drink and a snack to see him through till dinner. He wanted a bread roll and a banana with a glass of water. While he sat at the table eating, I set some toys in the living room together with my fostering folder, which contained my log notes, so I was ready for when Andrew arrived. I joined Oskar at the table with a mug of tea. Andrew knew we would be home by four o'clock and it was 4.30 now, so I was expecting him any time.

Oskar had just finished his snack when the doorbell rang. 'That'll be your social worker,' I said, standing.

He scrambled from his chair and, taking my hand, came with me to answer the front door.

'Hello,' Andrew said with a smile. 'How are you both?'

'Very well, thank you,' I replied.

'Shall I take off my shoes?' he asked, coming in and seeing ours paired in the hall.

'Yes, please, if you don't mind.' For hygiene and comfort we always take off our shoes when coming into the house, as do my extended family and friends, but some professionals don't, they march straight in, effectively using our carpets as a doormat. I find it disrespectful, although I rarely say anything.

'Would you like a drink?' I asked Andrew.

'Coffee, please.'

I showed him into the living room. Oskar was still holding my hand, so I gently eased it free and directed him to sit on the sofa. 'You can talk to Andrew while I make him a coffee,' I said. It was important Oskar got to know his social worker. 'Milk and sugar?' I asked Andrew.

'Just milk, please.'

I left the two of them sitting on the sofa while I went into the kitchen. Sammy came in through the cat flap, ignored me and went into the living room to see who was there. I heard him meow and then Andrew asked Oskar what the cat was called. 'Sammy,' Oskar replied. 'I'm allowed to feed him sometimes.'

I returned to the living room with Andrew's coffee, set it on the table within his reach and asked him if he wanted to speak to Oskar alone. It's usual for the social worker to spend some time alone with the child in case the child wants to raise something they don't feel comfortable saying in front of the foster carer. It's a strange feeling, being shut out in your own home, aware you are probably being talked about, but it's something foster carers have to get used to.

'You can stay for now,' Andrew said. 'Then I'll see Oskar alone later.' He took a sip of his coffee and I sat in one of the easy chairs opposite them, my fostering folder beside me, although many of the issues I needed to raise wouldn't be in front of Oskar.

'How are you settling in?' Andrew asked Oskar. Setting down his cup, he took a notepad and pen from his briefcase.

'OK,' Oskar said with his characteristic small shrug.

'Do you like having your own room?' Andrew asked, turning slightly so he could see him better.

'Yes,' Oskar said in a slight voice.

'I'll have a look at your bedroom before I leave,' Andrew said. 'Do you sleep well?'

Oskar shrugged.

'Surprisingly well so far,' I said.

'Good.' He made a note. 'What time does he go to bed?'

'We start his bath and bedtime routine at around seven o'clock, so he is usually asleep by eight. I wake him at seven to get ready for school.' Andrew was making notes. The social worker usually wanted to know the child's routine.

'And what about meals?' he asked Oskar. 'Do you have meals with the family?'

Oskar looked a bit unsure, so I said, 'We all have dinner together in the evening.'

'Are you having what you like to eat?' Andrew now asked him.

Oskar gave a small nod.

'He's eating well,' I said. 'He chose some rolls yesterday that he liked and he's been having those for breakfast. It would be useful to know what he eats at home with his mother and his likes and dislikes.'

Andrew wrote as he said, 'When his mother returns, I'll ask her.'

Oskar was now staring at his social worker at the mention of his mother, and Andrew saw this. 'I've spoken to your mother on the telephone,' he told him. 'She will see you when she comes back. She's with Luka now, but I think you know that, don't you?'

Oskar nodded.

'I've told your mother you are in foster care and are being well looked after. She is hoping to fly back this weekend if she can get a cheap flight. I'll arrange for you to see her next week and tell Cathy the details, all right?'

Oskar gave another small nod and Andrew took a sip from his coffee. Oskar's reaction to being told he would be seeing his mother next week was completely underwhelming and was very unusual for a child in care. Most children separated from their parent are ecstatic at the prospect of seeing them again.

'Do you have any questions?' Andrew asked him.

'How is Luka?' Oskar said.

'He's getting better and is back home with his aunt now.' Andrew then looked at me. 'Luka has cerebral palsy and is cared for by an aunt and her family. Oskar's mother, Roksana, works here and sends money to the aunt to look after Luka. He's been ill and had to go into hospital. Roksana wanted to see Luka and also had a money matter she needed to sort out.'

'I see,' I said. 'What a worry for her. Does Oskar see his brother?'

'Roksana said she takes him once a year at Christmas.' Oskar was nodding. 'Roksana can't afford to go home any more frequently, but as this was an emergency she scraped together the airfare for her to go and left Oskar at home with friends he calls aunts and uncles. The childcare arrangements are a bit complicated and it's something I'll be discussing with Roksana when she returns.'

'I see,' I said, and wondered if I might have done the two men waiting outside the school a disservice.

'Do you have any more questions?' Andrew asked Oskar.

He shook his head.

'Do you have everything you need to look after Oskar?' Andrew now asked me. It was a standard question asked by the child's social worker and my supervising social worker.

'Yes, although some more background information would be useful.'

'That reminds me,' he said, dipping his hand into his brief-case. 'I've got your copy of the placement forms.' He took them out and passed them to me. I tucked them into my fostering folder to read later.

'Your adult children live here too?' he asked me, glancing at the framed photographs of them on the walls.

'Yes. Adrian, Lucy and Paula. They'll be back shortly.'

Andrew made a note. 'And Oskar has age-appropriate self-care skills and is dry at night?'

'Yes.' It was another standard question; this type of information was needed for the report Andrew would write on his visit. He would also be observing Oskar in the placement and watching how he was settling in and relating to us – his foster family.

'If Oskar could have more of his toys from home that would be good,' I said.

'Yes, of course,' Andrew agreed as he wrote. 'I'll ask Roksana when she returns. But I can see you've got plenty of toys here in the meantime.'

I smiled. 'Yes, I've been fostering a long time.'

'What do you like playing?' Andrew now asked Oskar.

He shrugged.

'You did a jigsaw puzzle,' I prompted, but Oskar didn't add anything. 'I'm still trying to find out what interests him,' I told Andrew. 'He likes a bedtime story, but he's still wary of us all.'

It was only as I said this that I fully acknowledged just how true it was. Oskar was very wary around all of us, especially Adrian, more so than I would have expected or had experienced, and for reasons I couldn't identify.

'You like living here with Cathy and her family?' Andrew asked Oskar, who was still sitting impassively on the sofa beside him.

'Yes,' he said in the same small voice.

Andrew looked at him. 'What don't you like?'

Oskar didn't reply.

'Is this a good time for you to have a chat with him alone?' I asked Andrew.

'Probably,' Andrew said. 'Thank you.'

'I'm going to see to dinner,' I told Oskar as I stood.

He immediately looked anxious and was going to leave the sofa and come with me.

'You stay with Andrew,' I said. 'I'll be in the kitchen.'

'Just five minutes,' Andrew told him.

Oskar didn't look very reassured but stayed with Andrew as I left the room. It occurred to me that the only person Oskar seemed really comfortable with was his teacher, Miss Jordan. What, I wondered, or rather who, had made him so suspicious of adults by the age of six?

Drawing the living-room door closed behind me so Andrew and Oskar could talk in private, I went into the kitchen, put the casserole in the oven and then went into the front room and sat at my computer. Andrew had said five minutes, but once they got talking it would likely be longer and I tended to make the most of any free time I had. I opened the file I'd been working on, but no sooner had I done so than a key went in the front door as Paula let herself in.

'Hello, love,' I said. 'Oskar and his social worker are in the living room. Have you had a good day?'

'Yes,' she said. Slipping off her shoes and hanging her jacket on the hall stand, she came into the front room. I saved the file I was working on so we could talk.

A few minutes later the living-room door opened. 'Cathy?' Andrew called.

I went into the hall, and so too did Paula. Andrew and Oskar were standing at the far end.

'Oskar is a bit anxious and wants to know where you are,' Andrew said. Oskar actually smiled at Paula and looked pleased to see her, which was a first and positive.

'This is my youngest daughter, Paula,' I said, introducing her to Andrew.

'Hello. Pleased to meet you. Perhaps you can look after Oskar while I talk to your mother,' Andrew suggested.

'Yes, if he'll stay with me,' Paula said.

I went to Oskar. 'You can choose some games and puzzles from the toy cupboard and Paula will play with you while Andrew and I talk,' I told him. Apparently, Oskar preferred this option to having to stay with his social worker, and he went with Paula into our kitchen-diner where the toy cupboards are as Andrew and I returned to the living room. I now hoped to learn more about Oskar and have some of my questions answered.

CHAPTER SEVEN

VERY CONCERNED

'Oskar was very anxious with me,' Andrew said as he and I settled in the living room – him returning to the sofa and me to the easy chair where I'd left my fostering folder. 'It's his first time in care, so it's bound to take time for him to adjust.'

'Yes, indeed,' I agreed.

'I spoke to his mother, Roksana, at length on the phone yesterday,' Andrew continued. 'She's angry and upset Oskar is in foster care. As far as she's concerned, she made proper provision for him in her absence, and had no choice but to leave him with her friends. She says they were more than capable of looking after him and had done so in the past. She works long hours and they share childcare. She is adamant Oskar is always well looked after and that none of her friends would harm him. Has he said any more about the bruise on his cheek?'

'No, but he's not saying much to any of us at present, about anything.'

Andrew nodded and made a note. 'His mother says Oskar probably accidently banged his face and accused his uncle to gain sympathy in the hope she would come back. He didn't want her to go, but she says she had no choice and the uncle has looked after Oskar before.'

'Which uncle is this?' I queried.

'Mr Nowak, the one I met on Tuesday who came to collect Oskar from school.'

'Is this the same one Oskar is accusing of having hit him?'

'No. He wouldn't give that person's name to his teacher, but it's not Mr Nowak, or rather Uncle Nowak as Oskar calls him.'

'Are you aware there have been two other "uncles" waiting in a car outside the school?' I asked.

'No. When was this? I haven't had a chance to speak to the school since Tuesday when I placed Oskar.'

'They've been there each morning and afternoon, but the Headmistress spoke to them yesterday. They claimed they were family friends just keeping an eye on Oskar. I don't know their names. She asked them not to wait outside, as it was unsettling for Oskar, and I haven't seen them since.'

'I'll need to speak to the Head,' Andrew said, making a note.

'I raised it with the school because Oskar denied knowing them, although clearly he did and was very worried – almost frightened – by their presence. He didn't want to speak to them and was pleased to be in the school playground.'

Andrew nodded seriously as he wrote. 'Thanks.'

'If Oskar's mother was happy leaving him with friends, what did she have to say about all the times in the past when he's arrived at school hungry and grubby?' I asked.

'She says it's not true. The school have got it wrong. Although she admits she's not often there in the morning when Oskar gets up and leaves for school. She's a cleaner and starts work at six, as do most of the other women in the house. The men generally don't start work until later, so they are left in charge of the children and drop them off at school. Roksana often works the evening shift too, so whoever is available collects the children from school.'

'There are other children in the house?' I asked, concerned.

'Sometimes, and we're looking into that. You said on the phone that Oskar talked about three women who slept in the same room as him,' Andrew asked, checking his notes. 'Do you have their names?'

I opened my folder and read from my log notes. 'Maria, Elana and Alina. I don't have their surnames.'

'Thank you.' He wrote. 'Roksana is very upset that Oskar is now having to live with strangers. I've reassured her you are an experienced foster carer, but I thought it might help if she could meet you when she returns.'

'Yes, of course.' This request wasn't unusual. It's natural for a parent to want to meet the person who is looking after their child, and I would very likely be seeing her regularly at contact anyway.

'I'll arrange it once Roksana returns, and also set up supervised contact at the Family Centre,' Andrew continued. 'You will be able to take and collect him?'

'Yes.' It's a foster carer's duty to take the child to contact and then collect them afterwards. Sometimes they supervise contact too – in the community or at their own house – but this wasn't appropriate here. Oskar's contact would be observed by a specialist supervisor at the Family Centre.

'Did you have a chance to ask Oskar's mother about his diet and routine?' I asked Andrew.

'She confirmed Oskar has no special diet, or allergies, and eats most things. You can discuss his routine with her when you meet. She was very angry that he was in care, and also that he'd had a medical without her consent. I explained it was usual for a child to have a medical when they first come into care, and of course we didn't need her consent with the court order in place, although I would have sought it had she been here.' I nodded. 'I've read the paediatrician's report and she's noted Oskar is on the small side for his age but within the normal range. She couldn't find any other signs of non-accidental injury, although she states he was very reluctant to let her examine him.'

'Yes, he didn't want to remove his clothes. He doesn't want to undress in front of me, either. I run his bath and wait outside the door while he gets undressed and washes. Similarly, while he changes for bed. I wondered if it was what happened at home with so many in the house.'

'It's possible. I've yet to see the arrangements in the house, but it could be overcrowded. Oskar and his mother moved around quite a lot. Oskar's name has shown up on our system at various locations since he was eighteen months. He's attended two nurseries and three schools.'

'That is a lot,' I said. 'Although living here since he was little explains why his English is so good.'

'His mother would like them to settle here permanently, but it's complicated with Luka.' I nodded. 'She thought that once she returned Oskar could go to live with her again, so I've had to explain he will remain in care for the time being until all the checks are complete and we're satisfied he would be well looked after and not in any danger if he went home. She's not happy with me, but that's a social worker's lot, I'm afraid.' Andrew sighed resignedly.

I smiled sympathetically before asking, 'Did you know Oskar sleeps in a sleeping bag on the floor?'

'No,' he said, making a note. 'Has he told you that?'

'Yes, and also that he often gets into his sleeping bag in the evening and at weekends.'

'So he doesn't have a bed?' Andrew asked, frowning.

'Not according to him.'

'I'll be doing a home visit once Roksana is back, so I'll look at the sleeping arrangements then. I think that's all for now,' Andrew said, checking his notes. 'Do you have any further questions?'

'No, I don't think so.'

'I'll have a look around,' he said, returning his pad and pen to his briefcase, 'then I'll leave you to have your dinner. Something smells good.'

'That'll be the casserole,' I said. While we'd been talking the smell of the dinner cooking had drifted in from the kitchen.

As we stood, I heard the front door burst open and Lucy's excited cry of, 'Hi, guys! Guess what? Darren has finally seen the light. I've got a date tonight!'

'That's my other daughter, Lucy,' I told Andrew, and quickly stepped into the hall before she could say anything further. 'Hello, love, Oskar's social worker is here.'

'Whoops, I forgot!' Lucy said, clapping her hand over her mouth and grimacing. 'I hope he doesn't take me into care.'

'Lucy!' I cautioned. Andrew appeared in the hall.

'It's OK,' he said. 'I hope you have a nice evening.'

'Thanks,' she replied a little brusquely. 'I'm going to my room now to get ready.'

I smiled indulgently. Having been in and out of care herself for some years before coming to me, Lucy hadn't always had the best experience of social workers and had been quite anti them for a while. She was much better now, but could still be hostile sometimes, although I doubted she saw it that way, and I'm sure they'd experienced far worse.

I'd been about to show Andrew around our house, and I now led the way into our front room, which contained the desktop computer and printer we all used, bookshelves, a sound system, small sofa and an extending dining table with chairs that we used when we had guests. From there, I took him back down the hall and into the kitchen-diner, where Paula and Oskar were still at the table doing puzzles.

'Thank you,' I said to Paula, and I praised Oskar for playing nicely, as did Andrew.

I then showed Andrew upstairs, where he looked in all the rooms except Lucy's, as he said there was no need to disturb her. Sensible decision, I thought.

Downstairs again, Andrew collected his briefcase from the living room said goodbye to Oskar and Paula, and I showed him out. Five minutes later Adrian arrived home and I called everyone to dinner. Lucy joined us late, gobbled down her dinner and then returned to her room to finish getting ready, although I told her she looked beautiful as she was. Darren was a co-worker of hers at the nursery and she'd been talking about him for some time, so I'd known they were friends, but now it seemed their relationship had shifted to a different level. Adrian and Paula tempered and often internalized their feelings, but Lucy wore her heart on her sleeve. I was pleased she was going on a date but feared she might get hurt if she invested too much in their relationship too soon. But there is only so much you can say as a parent before advice becomes dogma.

Sometimes, when a child sees their social worker, it helps to reassure and settle them into their foster home, but Oskar was just as quiet and withdrawn after seeing Andrew as he had been before. He didn't mention his visit and I didn't press him, and so our evening continued. After dinner, Oskar and I went into the living room where he read his school book, then

I read him some stories before beginning his bath and bedtime routine. As on the previous evenings, I waited outside the bathroom door while he undressed, bathed and put on his pyjamas. Then I went in while he brushed his teeth. It was as we were going round the landing to his bedroom that he asked, 'Will I have to see Andrew again?'

'Yes, he's your social worker. If you have a problem, you can tell him or me.' Oskar frowned, worried. 'Andrew's nice,' I said. 'He wants to make sure you're safe and well looked after.'

He looked thoughtful and then asked, 'How do you know he's nice?'

'Because he's a social worker and wants to help children. He will have passed a lot of exams and checks to make sure he is suitable to work with children.'

Oskar went quiet again and as we entered his bedroom he asked, 'Is Adrian nice?'

'Yes, he's my son.'

Another thoughtful pause and then, 'Are my uncles nice?'

'I don't know, love. I've never met them. You probably know that better than me. What do you think?'

Silence. He picked up his teddy bear and, ignoring my question, said, 'My brother Luka is nice.'

'Yes, I'm sure he is. What about your uncles?' I asked.

Oskar climbed into bed and snuggled down on his side, facing away from me, signalling the conversation was over.

'Night, love, sleep tight,' I said. 'Friday tomorrow and then the weekend.'

There was no reply, so saying goodnight again, I came out, closing his bedroom door behind me.

* * *

In terms of fostering Oskar, I was having an easy time. Some children and young people arrive with huge behavioural problems and have passed through a number of foster carers before coming to me. Oskar was very well behaved, did as I asked, was eating and sleeping well, and was happy to go to school, but I wasn't reassured. His passive acceptance, the haunted look in his eye, his apparent wariness around men, and some of the questions he asked and statements he made but didn't follow through on gave me real cause for concern. My feeling that he had suffered more than neglect and a slap to his face increased, but it was still only a gut feeling from years of fostering; so far there was no evidence. When I wrote up my log notes that evening, I gave my usual objective account of Oskar's day, without any speculation or conjecture, but I was fearing the worse.

Lucy returned home from her date with Darren at around 10.30 p.m. I was in the living room, about to go up to bed, but she came in and wanted to talk. She was far less excitable now and looked tired – hardly surprising after a day at work and then all the energy that had gone into getting ready. She said she'd had a nice time, and as we talked I learnt that Darren was the same age as her, 23, and had a younger sister who already had a two-year-old child. Darren and their parents were very supportive.

'Good,' I said, while thinking I hoped Lucy had the sense not to go down the same route. 'Are you seeing him again?' I asked.

'Yes, tomorrow at work.'

'No, I meant on another date.'

'I hope so, I'd like to,' Lucy said. 'But he needs to do the running. I remember what you told me.'

'What was that, love?' I asked sceptically.

'You said, "Flee and they follow. Follow and they flee."'

I smiled weakly. 'Oh, yes, I remember, but don't take it too literally. That was the advice given back when I was courting John, and look where it got me!' John was my ex-husband.

'It's still true,' she said, taking my hand. 'Most guys like to do the running. It makes them feel in charge.'

'OK, if you say so. I'll look forward to meeting Darren.'

'Not yet, Mum!' she exclaimed, horrified. 'That's months away.'

Oskar slept well, dressed himself and then came down to breakfast and wanted his usual roll with a ham and cheese filling. When I eventually met his mother, I would ask her what else he liked for breakfast. I'd asked him a few times, but he had just shrugged. As in most instances like this, it was as if he didn't feel he had the right to voice his opinion or make choices but had to accept everything that came his way. Perhaps that was what had happened in the past.

At school there was no sign of the black car, although I saw Oskar looking. My friend Angela was in the playground again and came over to talk while we waited for the start of school. The children she was fostering played with their friends, while Oskar stayed close by my side. Once he'd gone into school I went home and phoned my mother to see if we could visit her at the weekend. She lived about an hour's drive away and I tried to see her most weekends. My father had died two years before. We also spoke on the phone a few times during the week. Mum was gentle, kind, patient, and she loved children. She and my father had always been very supportive of my fostering and I thought if anyone could persuade Oskar to relax and come out of his shell then she could.

CHAPTER EIGHT

PREOCCUPIED

Saturday was a more leisurely day for us all without any school, college or work. In the morning I set up various activities for Oskar to do at the table in the kitchen-diner and encouraged him to paint, model with dough, draw and play, all with some success. In the afternoon after lunch I took him to our local park, while Lucy, Adrian and Paula did what they wanted to at home. Paula had some college work to complete, and they were all going out later: Adrian to see his girlfriend, Kirsty, Paula with a friend to the cinema and Lucy on another date with Darren – preparations had already begun.

It was a fine spring day and there were plenty of other families in the park. I showed Oskar to the gated area where the children's play equipment was, but he didn't immediately run off to play as another child might. He stayed close beside me, apprehensive and wary. It took some encouragement to get him to try the apparatus, but eventually he began playing and, I think, enjoying himself in his own quiet way. As long as I was close at hand, he went from one piece of equipment to the next and played alongside the other children. I pushed him on the swings, spun the roundabout and then, as I rocked him on the sprung dragon, I asked casually, 'Does your mother take you to the park?'

'No, she works,' he replied.

'What about at weekends?'

'She works,' he said again.

'All of Saturday and Sunday?'

'Yes,' he replied. Lulled and occupied by the rocking motion, he was more willing to talk.

'So who looks after you at weekends?' I asked. No one was close enough to hear us.

'My aunts and uncles,' Oskar said.

'Do they take you out?'

'No. I stay in my sleeping bag.'

I doubted he did stay in his sleeping bag all weekend, but if he wasn't taken out it probably seemed like it. He was still enjoying the rocking dragon, so I continued to probe. 'Who cooks your meals at the weekends?'

'Whoever is in the house.'

'Your aunts and uncles?'

He nodded.

'Are they nice to you?'

Silence. He slowed the rocker and said, 'I want to play on something else.' His guard was up again and the moment had passed.

Once Oskar had exhausted all the play area had to offer, I took him to the duck pond on the other side of the park where a mother duck was swimming up and down, with her cute little ducklings following. I bought him an ice cream from the park café and we sat on a bench as he ate it. Then we took a slow walk back to the house and I thought Oskar was the most relaxed I'd seen him. He had some colour in his cheeks from being outside all afternoon and his expression was softer, less guarded. I'd found before that doing something together – even a small outing – can help a child relax, bond and feel part of the family. Although I didn't know how long Oskar would be with us, it was important he felt included and formed some attachment to us. I was therefore hoping that what had begun in the park would continue once we were home, allowing us to build on it.

However, as we began up our garden path the front door suddenly opened and Adrian stepped out, on his way to see Kirsty. Oskar started and I saw his expression change to one of caution and vigilance. It was the same reaction he'd had when he'd seen Andrew. I didn't think it had anything to do with them personally but suggested a wariness of men in general. Thankfully Adrian hadn't seen it and said, 'Hi, Oskar, did you have a good time in the park?'

Oskar gave a small nod, head down and chin pressed into his chest.

'Yes, thank you,' I said. 'Say hello to Kirsty. Will she be coming with us to Grandma's tomorrow?'

'No, she's seeing her own gran.'

'OK. Have a good evening. Give her my love.'

'Will do.' He kissed my cheek, said goodbye to us both and then disappeared down the path to his car.

As soon as Oskar and I were indoors I said, 'Adrian won't harm you, neither will Andrew.'

He concentrated on taking off his shoes.

'Most men are good like Andrew and Adrian, but there are a few who can hurt children. If that happens, it is important the child tells an adult they trust so the man can be stopped.' I thought that by putting it in general terms Oskar might feel able to tell me, but that wasn't going to happen yet. Having taken off his shoes and put on his slippers, he came with me into the kitchen where I began preparing dinner. He liked to be close by, so I gave him some little jobs to do and then he fed Sammy.

That evening, after we'd eaten and Paula and Lucy had gone out, I read to Oskar, then told him a little about my mother, who we were all going to see the following day, and where she lived. He sat quiet and accepting, as he was in most things. Once he was in bed, with the house to myself, I completed some work on my computer and then relaxed in the living room, where I watched a film on the television. I was in bed by the time Paula, Lucy and Adrian let themselves in. They were very quiet, but a short while later I heard the most appalling shriek from Oskar's room. Throwing on my dressing gown, I raced round the landing and, knocking on his door, went in. He was under the duvet, crying hysterically, 'No! Go away. Leave me alone.'

'Oskar,' I said kindly but firmly, turning up the light. 'It's Cathy.' I gently eased the duvet away from his face. His expression of horror and fear before he realized it was me was awful to see. 'Oskar, it's all right, love. You're safe. You're having a bad dream.' I sat on the edge of the bed and took him in my arms. He lay his head against my chest and sobbed.

I heard Paula's and Lucy's bedrooms doors open and they appeared on the landing outside Oskar's room, looking very worried. 'It's OK,' I told them. 'You go back to bed. I'll stay with him until he's settled.'

They returned to their rooms. I held Oskar and gently stroked his head, soothing him. 'You are safe. You had a bad dream.'

Eventually his sobbing eased, but his head still rested against me. 'Can you tell me what the dream was about?' I quietly asked him.

'No,' came his small reply.

'You're safe here in your own room,' I said. 'But if someone has hurt you in the past, it will help if you can tell me.'

'I want to go to sleep,' he said, changing the subject, and he drew away.

'All right.' He snuggled down, cuddling his teddy bear, and I drew the duvet over him.

'Can you close my door and leave my light on?' he asked from under the covers.

'Yes. But you are safe here,' I said again.

There was no reply, so, leaving the light on, I came out and closed his bedroom door as he'd asked. Of course, I could have believed the nightmare had simply been a product of Oskar's imagination, as bad dreams often are, had I not fostered abused children before whose only outlet for their past suffering was through night terrors.

Oskar didn't wake again and the following morning, Sunday, we all slept in a bit later – including Oskar. When I heard him moving around in his bedroom, I knocked on his door and went in. 'OK, love?'

He nodded, left his room to use the toilet and then returned to dress. 'You had a bad dream last night,' I said, setting out the clothes he would wear today to go to my mother's. 'Do you remember what it was about?'

'Yes,' he said quietly.

'Can you tell me?'

'No.' He began to dress, so I didn't ask any further questions at that point and left him to it.

* * *

At eleven o'clock we left the house to go to my mother's. Adrian drove my car and I sat in the passenger seat while Lucy and Paula sat in the rear with Oskar, keeping him amused with books and the iPad. Mum used to cook us all a traditional Sunday lunch when we visited her, but now she was in her eighties it had become too much, so I usually treated us to a meal out. I'd booked a table for today at a pub restaurant a short walk from where Mum lived. We'd been there before and it was child-friendly, with a small play area for children.

Mum must have been looking out for us, for as we pulled onto her driveway just before midday her front door opened and there she stood, ready to greet us, smiling and waving. She always makes such a fuss of us and the children we foster. Although I'd left home many years before when I'd married, it still felt as though I was coming home each time I visited. As we filed in, Mum kissed us one by one and I introduced Oskar. 'Would you like a kiss?' she asked him, but he shook his head. She understood. 'Another time then, when you know me better. I'll show you where the toys are.'

Mum keeps a large toy box for the children in the living room, but Oskar wasn't going anywhere without me. Holding his hand, I took him through to the living room and then sat on the floor with him and encouraged him to explore the toy box. Lucy and Paula had gone into the kitchen with Mum to make us some drinks. Adrian was with them too, asking Mum if she had any odd jobs she needed doing. Since my father had died, Adrian did the general maintenance jobs that my father had done; for example, cutting the grass and clearing a blocked gutter. My brother and his family helped out too.

There was nearly an hour before we needed to leave for the restaurant so we sat in Mum's living room with our drinks. I would like to say that Oskar quickly relaxed around Mum – or rather Nana, as most of the children we fostered called her – and was soon following her around as he did me. But that wasn't so. He remained watchful and on high alert. Every noise that came from inside or outside the house startled him and he anxiously looked to see where it had come from. It got a bit easier as we walked to the pub restaurant and during lunch, perhaps because we were in neutral territory, I don't know, but once we returned he sat by me for the rest of the afternoon. When it was time to go, Mum said to me, 'Oskar seems a nice child, but he's far too quiet.'

'I know. Hopefully he'll be more at ease next time we visit.'

On Monday morning, Edith, my supervising social worker (SSW), telephoned. She asked how Oskar was settling in and said she wanted to visit us the following afternoon. I told her we would be home from school by four o'clock and then made a note in my diary that she was coming. An hour later Andrew telephoned. He asked how Oskar was and then said, 'Oskar's mother, Roksana, is due back in the UK tomorrow evening. I'm going to see her Wednesday morning, and I'll set up a meeting for you to meet her in the afternoon at two o'clock. I'll also arrange supervised contact for Oskar to see his mother on Wednesday at the Family Centre, four o'clock until five-thirty.'

'OK.' I reached for my diary and scribbled down these arrangements. 'Where am I meeting Roksana?' I asked as I wrote.

'Here at the council offices.'

'I'll need to leave at three o'clock to collect Oskar from school and take him to the Family Centre,' I said.

'That should be fine. It's just a short, informal meeting.'

'Do you want me to tell Oskar he will be seeing his mother?' I asked.

'Yes, please. I won't have a chance before.'

We said goodbye. My diary was quickly filling. I had Edith visiting straight after school on Tuesday afternoon, the meeting with Roksana on Wednesday, followed by contact, and a day's foster-carer training on Thursday.

That afternoon, when I collected Oskar from school, I told him what his social worker had said: that his mother was returning tomorrow so he would be able to see her on Wednesday at the Family Centre. Most children would have been ecstatic at the prospect of seeing their mother again, but not Oskar.

'Yes,' he said, his voice flat.

I explained a bit about the Family Centre. 'It's like a big house with lots of living rooms,' I said as I drove. 'You will see your mother in one of the rooms. It has a sofa, table and chairs, and lots of games and toys.' All the rooms used for contact were similar. 'Other children will be seeing their families in the other rooms too. A lady called a contact supervisor will be with you the whole time to make sure you're all right.'

'Yes,' he said in the same voice. I appreciated it was a lot for him to take in.

'In the past I've taken many other children I've looked after to the Family Centre,' I continued. 'They always had a good time with their parents.'

He didn't reply.

'Oskar, are you happy you are seeing your mother?' I asked, glancing at him in the rear-view mirror.

'Yes,' he said in a tone that suggested he wasn't. He changed the subject. 'I've got maths homework in my school bag.'

'OK. I'll help you with it after dinner. Is there anything worrying you?' I glanced at him in the rear-view mirror. He shook his head. 'You know you can tell me if there is.'

He didn't reply and the subject of contact, the Family Centre and seeing his mother wasn't mentioned again.

As it turned out, Oskar didn't need my help with his homework, but I sat with him at the table anyway while he completed it, then I heard him read. Afterwards, he watched some television, quietly and not really engaged with the programme, as he often seemed to be – gazing into the distance with a slight frown. At seven o'clock we followed our usual bedtime routine.

The following morning, Miss Jordan came into the playground as Oskar and I waited for the start of school and made a point of asking me how he was settling at my house. 'Slowly,' I said. 'How is he at school?'

'He does his work nicely but seems preoccupied,' she said, lowering her voice.

'I know exactly what you mean,' I agreed. Preoccupied summed up Oskar perfectly. Most of the time I had the feeling he was there in body, while his thoughts were a million miles away. 'He's seeing his mother after school tomorrow,' I told her. It's important the child's teacher knows of any events that could impact on their general well-being and learning, so they can make allowances and offer support if necessary. I remember going into my children's school when my husband left me and telling the Head. My children didn't need additional support to get them through what was a very difficult time for us all, but it was reassuring to know it was there if necessary.

Oskar was standing by my side as Miss Jordan and I talked, and she now spoke to him. 'I expect you're pleased to be seeing your mother again.'

'Yes,' Oskar said, without any indication of being pleased.

'There's a lot to adjust to,' I told her. 'What was their relationship like before?' I asked quietly.

'It's difficult to say. He was usually dropped off and collected by his uncles. Will he be seeing her regularly?'

'Yes, I would think so. His social worker will give me the details.'

'What about his uncles? Will he be seeing some of them?'

'Not as far as I know.'

Edith's visit that afternoon was predictable if nothing else. In my experience, supervising social workers can interpret their role differently. My previous SSW, Jill, was very hands-on, committed and enthusiastic, often going beyond the call of duty or her job description. Edith, on the other hand, was more reserved in her energy and passion for the job, but we got along.

She arrived half an hour late, didn't apologize or remove her shoes and, saying a rather curt hello to Paula who'd just come home, took herself through to the living room where Oskar was patiently waiting for her. 'How are you?' she asked quite brusquely, sitting next to him.

'OK,' he said quietly, and moved further along the sofa.

'Have you been to school?' she asked in the same tone.

He didn't reply.

'Has he been to school?' she asked me, taking a notepad and pen from her shoulder bag.

'Yes.'

'Is he seeing his family?'

'He is seeing his mother tomorrow.'

While she was writing, Oskar slipped quietly from the sofa and left the room. I heard him go up to his bedroom. 'Oh, he's gone,' she said. 'Never mind. I've seen him.'

The rest of Edith's visit followed its usual course. The outline is the same for most SSWs; it's the interpretation that's different. She gave me a copy of her report from her last visit, which I had to read, sign and return – I'd be emailed a copy for my records. Then, making notes as I replied, she asked questions from her check list: what were the contact arrangements? I didn't know yet. How was Oskar doing at school? I told her. Were there any placement issues or changes in my household? No. Was Oskar receiving his pocket money? Yes. How much was I saving for him? 'Ten pounds a week,' I replied. All carers are expected to save for the child they are looking after. Edith then asked what training I'd attended since her last visit, made a note, and then read and signed my log notes. She looked around the house, called goodbye to Oskar, who was still in his bedroom, and left to write her report on this meeting. She'd done her job, but I never felt there was any real involvement or warmth.

That evening Oskar was even quieter than normal, if that were possible. I asked him if he was all right and he nodded. I asked him if he was nervous about seeing his mother tomorrow. He shrugged, so I reassured him there was nothing to worry about. However, that night he had another nightmare and when I went to his room, he murmured, only half awake, 'Am I seeing Mummy at my house?'

'No, at the Family Centre,' I replied, settling him. Reassured, he went straight back to sleep.

CHAPTER NINE

A STRANGE REUNION

While Oskar wasn't showing any emotion at seeing his mother again, I was pretty churned up and nervous inside. It's always worrying, meeting the child's family for the first time, wondering if they are going to like me and hoping we can get along. It is important for the child to see their parent(s) and carer(s) working together, but it's not always possible. Some parents remain very angry that their child is in care and direct it at the carer, constantly criticizing them and fault-finding, trying to undermine their role, even to the point of making unfounded allegations. Hopefully, Roksana wouldn't be like that and we could work together for Oskar's sake.

I changed into a smart outfit for our meeting. Andrew was seeing Roksana that morning, I assumed at her house. Hopefully, he had been able to reassure her that Oskar was being well looked after so she would be calmer and more accepting by the time we met.

I arrived at the council offices five minutes early, signed in at reception and then asked the receptionist which room the meeting was in. She didn't have it listed but spent some time phoning various extensions, trying to find out where I should go, before calling Andrew's mobile. He told her the meeting was in Room 7 and he was already there. I thanked her for her trouble and, looping the Visitor's Pass around my neck, went up the stairs to Room 7.

Andrew and the woman I assumed to be Roksana were sitting on the opposite side of a large table. Roksana was well built with brown hair and a pale complexion, but her eyes were red from crying. There was a plastic cup of water and a box of tissues on the table in front of her and she'd just been about to reach for another tissue when, on seeing me, she abruptly stood and rushed towards me. For a moment I thought she was going to hit me. I think Andrew did too, because he stood. But Roksana didn't lash out, far from it. She threw her arms around me and sobbed, 'Please, you must help me get my child back! He's all I've got.'

I'd met many parents before who'd been upset, but not one who dissolved into tears on my shoulder at our first meeting. I was deeply moved as she wept openly. 'You must help me, please. Oskar is my reason for living,' she said, distraught.

I'll admit I felt slightly uncomfortable at the close physical contact of this stranger, but I couldn't just ease her away. Andrew was looking at us awkwardly, clearly not sure what to do for the best as Roksana continued to cry. 'I'm so sorry I went away. I had to go for my other child, but I promise I won't do it again.' She had a slight accent, which seemed to highlight her emotion and remorse.

I comforted her as best I could and presently Andrew picked up the box of tissues and came over. 'Shall we sit down?' he asked, offering her the tissues.

Roksana took one and wiped her eyes. 'Sorry,' she said, regaining control, and we sat at the table.

'I know it's difficult,' I said to her.

'Thank you,' she said, and blew her nose. 'I'm embarrassed, but it's all such a shock. I had to see my other son, Luka – he's not well – but now I've lost Oskar. I haven't seen him for nearly three weeks.'

'You're seeing him this afternoon,' I said, and Andrew nodded. I knew this wasn't much by way of reassurance, but it was all I could think of.

'Thank you for looking after Oskar,' she said without any resentment.

I felt so sorry for her. Andrew was still looking awkward and I wondered how their meeting that morning had gone; it had probably been more difficult than this one. She took a sip of water.

'Roksana feels she has been treated unfairly,' Andrew now said, looking at me. 'And it was unnecessary for us to apply for a care order. I've explained our reasons and have suggested she takes legal advice.'

'I have an appointment with a solicitor tomorrow,' Roksana said. 'But I don't have enough money for a lawyer. Andrew says I will be given help.'

'I believe you can apply for legal aid,' I said.

'Do you remember, I gave you some literature?' Andrew reminded her.

She nodded. 'I haven't read it yet.'

'Your solicitor will be able to explain more about legal aid, and how to apply,' Andrew said. Roksana looked lost and I appreciated what a daunting and massive task it must seem to a parent whose child had been taken into care, to have to deal with the legal complexities of the care system while grieving for their child. However, I reminded myself that if Oskar hadn't been badly treated and in danger he would never have been taken into care. It had been done to protect him.

'I didn't hurt him,' Roksana blurted out, as if reading my thoughts. 'And neither did any of my friends.'

'I think it might help if you could tell Roksana a bit about yourself and how Oskar is doing,' Andrew said to me, changing the subject. We only had an hour and we were already twenty minutes into it.

'Yes, of course.'

'In my country we pay people to look after children,' Roksana said. 'And they're not always nice to them.'

'We have high standards of foster care here,' Andrew said, and looked to me to continue.

'I have been fostering for a long time – over twenty-five years – and I always do the best I can for the child I'm looking after,' I began.

'Do they all go home?' she interrupted.

'Not in all cases,' I replied honestly, hoping I was saying the right thing. 'But those who can't are found permanent loving homes.'

'*I* love Oskar,' she said forcefully. 'My home is good.'

I nodded and continued. 'I am divorced and have three grown-up children who live with me, a son and two daughters. The children we look after are always treated as part of our family. Oskar has his own bedroom and I have plenty of toys and games for him to play. We eat together whenever possible and I have been taking him to school and helping him with his homework.'

'Do you take him to school every day?' she asked.

'Yes, and meet him. If for any reason I can't then my daughters, Lucy and Paula, are my nominated carers and they can help if necessary.'

'Yet I am in trouble for letting others help me and take Oskar to school!' she shot back, annoyed. I could see her point.

86

'My daughters have been assessed as being suitable and are police-checked,' I replied.

'What does "police-checked" mean?'

'Their details are run through a database to make sure they don't have any criminal convictions,' I said. 'All members of a foster carer's family are police-checked.'

I saw a flash of recognition, guilt maybe, possibly suggesting she or someone who was responsible for Oskar could have a criminal record. But that wasn't for me to comment on. The social services would look into it. I continued to describe my house, a typical day and what we liked to do in our leisure time, including activities especially for Oskar. I then asked, 'If you could tell me what sort of things Oskar likes, and his routine, it would help me look after him.'

'Routine?' she asked.

'Yes, you know, when he goes to bed and gets up. If he prefers a shower or a bath in the morning or evening. What he likes to do in the evenings and weekends. That sort of thing.'

'I don't know. I work long hours. My friends take care of him. You'll have to ask them.'

I was surprised by her admission that she didn't know her child's routine, but she seemed unfazed.

'It doesn't matter,' I said. 'I have established a routine, but I always try to include the parents' wishes if possible. Do you know what Oskar likes to eat?'

'Most things,' she said. 'He has what he is given.'

I nodded. I saw Andrew watching her carefully.

'He chose some rolls for breakfast and he's been having them with a cheese and ham filling,' I said. 'Is there anything else he might like?'

'Breakfast is not a big meal for us. We all have to leave for work, so a roll or bread with butter and jam is OK.'

'And for the evening you are happy for him to have what we have? It's usually meat or fish and vegetables, casseroles, stews, sometimes pasta, that sort of thing.'

'Yes, he has what we do. There are no special meals for children.'

I nodded. 'Is there anything Oskar really doesn't like?'

'I don't think so.'

'And he doesn't have any allergies?'

'No. Andrew asked me that.'

'I've bought Oskar new clothes, but if there is anything you want him to have from home, can you send them, please? Also, any of his toys.'

'There was no need for you to buy new clothes,' Roksana said indignantly. 'He has plenty. I work hard to buy him clothes, but my friend didn't pack them for you. I was angry when I found out. I can send more.'

'It's not a problem,' I said. 'But if you would like Oskar to have them, that's fine.'

'Perhaps you can take them to contact this afternoon,' Andrew suggested to Roksana.

'I won't have time to go home this afternoon, but I will bring them another time.'

'Good, thank you,' I said. 'It'll be nice for him to have his own belongings. Are there any toys he might like to have with him?'

'Maybe. I'll have a look in his sleeping bag,' she replied.

'Is that where Oskar keeps his toys?' I asked. 'Oskar mentioned a sleeping bag.'

'Yes. The children keep their toys in their sleeping bags so they don't get lost.'

'Everyone in the house has their own sleeping bag on a mattress on the floor,' Andrew explained. I assumed he'd seen this when he'd visited Roksana at home that morning.

'Do the children sleep in their sleeping bags as well?' I asked.

'Yes,' Roksana said. 'They are easy to store and if we have to move quickly or go home, we can pack them easily.'

I nodded. I could see the logic in this, and it confirmed what Oskar had told me, but whether this sleeping arrangement would meet the approval of the social services was another matter. If there was any chance of Oskar eventually returning home, the social services would need to be satisfied he wasn't in any danger and his needs were being met. The parenting didn't have to be perfect, just 'good enough'. It is a recognized term in child-care proceedings that requires the child's health and developmental needs are always put first by providing a routine and consistent care.

'My friends have been looking after Oskar,' Roksana now said. 'There was no need for you to take him to the doctor.' I assumed she was referring to the medical.

Andrew answered. 'Most children have a medical when they first come into care,' which I guessed he'd already told her.

'And the doctor said he was healthy?' she asked me.

'Yes, although she thought he was quiet, as he has been with me.'

'Oskar is always quiet. He is a good boy,' she said defensively. 'He never gives me any trouble. I have brought him up to do as he is told. So if the doctor says he is well, he can come home?' she asked Andrew, clearly not understanding the process.

'Not yet. We have assessments to make,' Andrew replied. 'Your solicitor will explain. Is there anything else you would like to ask Cathy? I'm mindful of the time.'

'You have a house just for you and your family?' she asked me.

'Yes.'

She frowned and looked at Andrew. 'But I can't afford to rent a house for me and Oskar. After I have paid for Luka's care, I have nothing left. I have to share a house.'

'You don't need a house,' Andrew confirmed. 'Perhaps we could talk about this after? Is there anything else you want to ask Cathy?'

Roksana shook her head, a little like Oskar did.

'Cathy, anything you want to add?' Andrew asked me.

I looked at Roksana. 'I was wondering if you have a photograph of you and Luka that Oskar could have in his bedroom while he is with me. Children find it comforting to have a photo of their family.'

She frowned, puzzled. 'I have one of Luka on my phone, as I don't see him often. But I see Oskar, and soon he will be living with me again.'

My heart went out to her. She had very little understanding of the care system and what lay ahead. I didn't think it was Andrew's fault for not explaining. Like many parents whose children are suddenly taken into care without any warning she'd gone into panic mode and wasn't understanding or listening to what she was being told. Probably blotting it out in a bid to cope. 'My lawyer will make it OK,' she added quietly.

With the meeting at an end, I told Roksana that I would see her at the Family Centre at four o'clock for contact and that I had to go now to collect Oskar from school. 'I'll come with you,' she said. 'It's a long way for me on the bus.'

I knew Andrew wouldn't consider that appropriate at this stage in the proceedings. 'I'll take you to the Family Centre in my car today,' he offered. 'Then in future you can catch a bus or take a cab.'

'I haven't the money for a cab,' she replied anxiously.

'The department should be able to give you some help with that,' he said.

I said goodbye and left Andrew reassuring Roksana that help could be given with transport so she could see Oskar.

'Am I seeing Mummy?' Oskar asked as soon as he came out of school.

'Yes, we're going there now.'

However, instead of being pleased, he immediately became sullen.

'You'll have a nice time,' I said as we left the playground. There was no response.

As I drove, I made light conversation by asking him about his day at school, as I usually did.

'Have you had a good day?'

'OK,' he replied.

'What subjects did you have?'

'Science.'

'You like science. What did you learn?'

He shrugged.

'What else did you do?'

'Don't know.'

'Did you have a nice lunch?' I asked, glancing at him in the rear-view mirror. I saw him shrug again. 'Oskar, is everything all right?'

Silence.

'Are you worrying about seeing your mother?'

'No.'

'Has that car been outside your school again?'

'No.'

'Please tell me if anything is worrying you and I will do my best to help.'

I drew up and parked outside the Family Centre and opened Oskar's car door. He clambered out and slipped his hand into mine as we went up the path to the security-locked main door, where I pressed the buzzer. The closed-circuit television camera overhead allowed anyone in the office to see who was at the door. After a moment, the door clicked open and we went in. I said hello to the receptionist who was sitting at her computer behind a low security screen to our right, and then I signed the Visitors' Book. I knew the procedure from bringing children here before to see their families.

'Has Roksana arrived yet?' I asked the receptionist.

'Yes. The social worker is here too. They are in Green Room.'

I thanked her, and with Oskar holding my hand again we went through the double doors and along the corridor towards Green Room. The six rooms in the centre are referred to by the colour they are decorated. The door to Green Room was slightly open, so I knocked and we went in. Andrew was standing with Roksana in the centre of the room, and he was the one who greeted us. 'Hello, Oskar, Cathy. I'll be staying for a little while.' It wasn't unusual for the social worker to stay at the first contact, and then they usually observed it from time to time.

The contact supervisor was already sitting at the table with a large notebook open in front of her. Roksana would have had her role explained when she was shown around the Family Centre, so she should have been aware she was taking notes. Whether Roksana knew her report would be sent to

Andrew, who would incorporate it in his final report to the judge, was a different matter. Ultimately, what the contact supervisor wrote would be taken into consideration when the judge made their decision on whether Oskar was allowed home. I feel for parents in this position, being continually observed, but there is little alternative if contact needs to be supervised because of safeguarding issues.

I was now expecting Roksana and Oskar to fall into each other's arms, hugging, kissing and probably crying with joy at seeing each other again after so long, as I'd witnessed so many families do in the past. They hadn't seen each other for three weeks and their emotions must be running high. Roksana had been very upset at our meeting earlier and I was anticipating that Oskar, who'd been keeping a tight lid on his emotions, would finally let his guard drop and run to his mother.

It didn't happen.

Roksana remained where she was and Oskar continued to stand by my side, holding my hand and looking warily at his mother from across the room. She looked back, equally warily. 'Hello, Oskar,' she said, her voice flat. 'How are you?'

I looked at him, expecting him to drop my hand and go to her, but again, neither of them moved. Andrew was watching this strange interaction too, as was the contact supervisor, who would doubtless note it.

Normally, once I've seen a child into the contact room, I leave, as it is their time with their parent(s), but it was clear mother and son needed some help.

'Come on, let's find some games for you and your mother to play,' I said to Oskar. I drew him to the shelves and cupboards where all the toys were. Roksana was still watching him, as were Andrew and the contact supervisor.

'Look, here are some jigsaw puzzles. You like doing those,' I said. I slid some boxes from the shelves and placed them on the coffee table in front of the sofa. I thought that once they got playing they would feel less awkward. Neither of them moved. 'I'll see you at five-thirty then,' I said.

Andrew was the only one who replied. 'Yes.'

I said goodbye and left. The silence followed me out. It was the strangest, eeriest, coldest reunion I had witnessed in all my years of fostering.

CHAPTER TEN

CONTACT

Whatever had happened between Roksana and Oskar to make them so cautious of each other? I wondered as I drove home from the Family Centre. It wasn't normal. Having been separated for three weeks, neither of them had anything to say to each other and apparently felt nothing on being reunited. Or possibly they had felt plenty, but for whatever reason weren't able to show their emotions, with neither willing to make the first move. Hopefully they were getting along better now.

I had just enough time to go home for half an hour before I had to leave to return to the Family Centre to collect Oskar. Paula arrived home while I was there and I left her instructions on when to put the fish pie I'd made earlier into the oven so it would be ready for dinner.

I arrived at the Family Centre five minutes early, signed the Visitors' Book and then waited in the corridor. I knew that every minute was precious to families who are separated, so I never interrupted before their time was up. As I waited, I could hear children's voices coming from other contact rooms and a baby crying. At exactly 5.30 p.m. I continued along the corridor to Green Room. The door was closed, so I knocked and went in. The silence hit me.

Andrew had gone, the contact supervisor was at the table, writing, and Oskar and his mother were sitting side by side on the sofa, close but not touching. I assumed that whatever they'd been playing with had been packed away, for clearly they hadn't just been sitting there for one and a half hours.

As soon as Roksana saw me she stood and began putting on her coat. 'Good, you're here,' she said intensely. 'Can you give me a lift to work? I'm going to be late.' Oskar remained sitting on the sofa.

'I'm sorry, I can't today,' I said. 'I'll need Andrew's permission and he won't be in the office now. We can ask him tomorrow and perhaps I can help you out next time.'

She tutted, picked up her handbag and threw it over her shoulder, clearly stressed at being late for work.

'I'm sorry,' I said again. 'I'll ask Andrew, although if you explain the problem to him he may be able to alter the times of contact to fit around your work.'

'I have to rush,' she said and, throwing a kiss at the top of Oskar's head, called goodbye as she ran out the door. Oskar stayed where he was on the sofa.

I would have liked to help her, but if she and Oskar were in my car it would have constituted a form of contact, so I needed Andrew's permission. I knew that Roksana worked as a cleaner in various offices, and if they were on my way and Andrew agreed then I'd been happy to drop her off next time. Alternatively, as I'd suggested to her, contact arrangements might be adjusted to fit around her work, although the centre was only open from 9.00 a.m. to 5.30 p.m., Monday to Friday. I appreciated it was difficult for parents who worked full-time, but seeing their children was usually a priority.

Oskar stood, picked up his jacket and came to me, tucking his hand into mine. I gave it a reassuring squeeze said goodbye to the contact supervisor, and we left. 'Did you have a nice time?' I asked Oskar as we walked down the corridor.

He shrugged.

'Did you play some games with your mother?' I tried.

'Yes.'

'Good.' I signed out of the Visitors' Book. 'What did you play?'

'The games you got from the shelf.'

'Anything else?'

'I can't remember. What's for dinner?'

'Fish pie and green beans.'

Usually when I collected a child from contact they were brimming over with excitement, wanting to tell me what a fantastic time they'd had with their parents and then counting off the days until their next contact. Oskar didn't mention seeing his mother all evening, and his reaction was worrying. I hoped I would be given some feedback from the contact. My experience in the past was that this was sporadic. Sometimes the social worker passed on feedback and other times they didn't. It's very useful if the foster carer is given a brief résumé of what happened in contact so we are better able to deal with any issues that may arise from it or questions the child might ask.

After dinner, when there was just Oskar and me in the living room, I asked him, 'Were you happy to see your mother?' For I really didn't know.

'Yes,' he said, but his face was expressionless, as it often was.

'Are you happy to see her again?' I asked. It wouldn't be his decision, but it was important we knew his feelings.

'Yes, but she has to work,' he replied, his voice flat.

'I know, but she and Andrew can make some arrangements that suit her. It's important you see each other, isn't it?'

'Is it?' he asked.

97

I hid my shock. Most children would know how important it was to see their parents.

'I think so. She loves you, and you love her, don't you?'

'Yes, but she has to work,' he said again. 'Can I go to bed? I'm tired.' Which was Oskar's way of telling me he didn't want to talk about his mother any more. But then he never wanted to talk about her.

I read him a bedtime story and took him up for his bath. That night I asked him – as I had been doing every night – if he wanted a goodnight kiss. To my surprise, he gave a small nod. 'Here, like Mummy did,' he said, pointing to the top of his head. I knew then how much that fleeting goodbye kiss from his mother had meant to him.

'Does your mother kiss you goodnight?' I asked.

'No, she's at work.'

'What about your aunts and uncles?'

He shook his head.

'So who sees you into bed?'

'No one. I have a wash and get into my sleeping bag.'

A lump rose to my throat at the image of little Oskar, so young and vulnerable, taking himself off to his sleeping bag every night without a loving goodnight kiss or hug. 'Do you want a hug as well?' I asked as he snuggled down, but he shook his head shyly. I kissed the top of his head and, saying goodnight, came out and closed the door. It would be another month before he wanted a hug.

The following morning, the Guardian ad Litem (or Guardian as they are often referred to in child-care proceedings) telephoned me. Tamara Hastings had also been the Guardian for the two children I'd looked after just before Oskar and whose story I tell in *Innocent*.

'I thought I recognized your name,' she said. 'How are you?'

'Very well, thank you, and you?'

'Yes, good. How is Oskar settling in?'

I told her more or less what I'd told Andrew, so she was up to date. We didn't discuss the previous case as it wouldn't have been appropriate. The Guardian is usually a qualified social worker and is appointed by the court in child-care proceedings for the duration of the case. They are independent of the social services but have access to all the files. They see all parties involved in the case, including the children, their parents and social services, and report to the judge on what is in the best interests of the child. The judge usually follows their recommendation.

Once I'd finished updating her, she made an appointment to visit us after school the following Monday. I noted it in my diary.

Andrew telephoned that afternoon and asked how Oskar had been after contact. He said he had stayed for half an hour and had also spoken to the contact supervisor this morning. I said Oskar had been quiet but that wasn't unusual, and when I asked him what he and his mother had done he said they'd played with some board games. I then paraphrased the rest of what Oskar had said, including his comments about his mother working.

'It appears that Roksana has always worked very long hours,' Andrew said. 'It may have impacted on their relationship. I appreciate that supervised contact isn't a natural environment, but Roksana struggled to relate to her son and he to her. The contact supervisor said that Roksana was very worried about being late for work and mentioned this a few times, which worried Oskar.'

'Yes, he told me that. I think Roksana is going to ask you about changing the times of contact.'

'I haven't spoken to her yet today, but I'm proposing contact will be three times a week, four to five-thirty. I've left a message on her voicemail to phone me. I think she's seeing her solicitor this afternoon. If you don't hear from me, assume the next contact will be on Friday at four o'clock.'

I made a note. 'Roksana asked me if I could give her a lift to work after contact. I told her she'd need to speak to you first.'

'OK, I'll talk to her and let you know. Has Oskar said anything about his uncle hitting him?'

'No.'

'The contact supervisor said Roksana told Oskar not to say bad things about his uncles.'

'I see. No, he hasn't said anything to me.'

'OK. Thank you.'

Roksana should have known better than to say that at contact. One of the reasons contact is supervised when there has been an allegation of abuse and care proceedings are current is to stop a parent threatening or coercing their child into withdrawing an allegation. Roksana wasn't doing herself any favours.

An hour later Andrew telephoned again. I was now in the playground, waiting for the end of school. I moved away from the others so I couldn't be overheard.

'I've spoken to Roksana,' Andrew said. 'Because of her work commitments she can only see Oskar on Tuesday and Thursday for an hour – from four to five. Then she has to start the evening shift. I've checked with the Family Centre and there is a room free then. She has asked for phone contact on the other days, which I have agreed to, but I would like you to supervise it, so put your phone on speaker.'

'All right. When does this new arrangement begin?'

'Start the phone contact this evening, and then they will see each other next Tuesday and Thursday. Do you have Roksana's mobile number?'

'Yes, it's in the placement information forms. What time should Oskar phone her?' I asked.

'Between five and five-thirty is good for her, or after ten, but I'm guessing Oskar will be in bed by then.'

'Yes, he goes up around seven. And the lift home she wanted?'

'It won't be necessary with these new arrangements.'

'OK.'

I ended the call with a heavy heart. A parent who was fighting to get their child back should be demanding more contact, not less. Andrew had offered Roksana three ninety-minute sessions a week and she'd cut it to two sessions of an hour each. Yes, she had to work and she was gaining phone contact, but it wouldn't be viewed in a positive light. The inference could be drawn that if Roksana wasn't able to make time to see her child while he was in care then she was unlikely to have the time to successfully parent him if he was returned to her.

I obviously didn't tell Oskar this when he came out of school. I began by asking him if he'd had a good day, and he replied, 'Yes. I like school.'

'Excellent.'

As we walked to the car I told him I'd spoken to Andrew and then explained the new contact arrangements in a positive light. 'So you will be seeing your mother twice a week and speaking to her on the phone on the other days,' I said.

'Will I have to speak to my uncles?' he asked quietly.

'No. Just your mother.' I unlocked the car door. 'Why? Do you want to speak to your uncles?'

'No.'

Before I started the engine, I swivelled round in my seat so I could see Oskar. 'I've looked after a lot of children,' I said. 'And I get a sense when something is wrong. If there is anything worrying you, I think it would help if you could tell me.'

He shrugged.

'I know when you saw Mummy yesterday she asked you not to talk about when your uncle slapped you, but it is important you tell.'

'He did slap me!' Oskar blurted. 'I told Miss Jordan the truth.'

'Yes, I believe you, so did she.'

'Mummy doesn't,' he said, his face falling. 'She thinks I made it up.'

'I know, it's difficult for her. Why do you think she would say that?' I asked.

'Because I don't like being left alone with those men. Some are nice, but others aren't.' It was the most Oskar had said and I wanted to learn as much as possible before he clammed up again.

'Which men are nice?' I asked.

'Uncle Nowak.'

'Anyone else?'

'Some are OK.'

'Who isn't nice?'

Silence.

'Do you know their names?'

102

He looked thoughtful and then shook his head. 'I can't remember.'

'OK. If you do, tell me, please.'

Andrew had said we should telephone Roksana between 5.00 and 5.30, so shortly after 5.00, with Oskar sitting beside me, I made the call, blocking the caller identity on my landline. Roksana wasn't to be given my contact details. It went through to voicemail, so I left a message. 'Hello, it's Cathy, Oskar's carer. Andrew said to phone. I'll call you back in ten minutes.' I knew that many people didn't answer their phones if the number was withheld. I explained this to Oskar.

Ten minutes later I called again and Roksana answered straight away. 'It's Cathy. Oskar is here, ready to talk to you.'

'Andrew said you were going to listen in,' she said. 'Are you recording this call?'

'No, it's just on speakerphone. Only Oskar and I are present.'

I passed the phone to Oskar. I'd had to supervise phone contact before and it's never easy to begin with. I felt uncomfortable listening in and obviously it's not nice for the parents, but this was worse than most. I didn't know if it was the fact that Roksana knew I was listening or whether their conversation would have been stilted anyway, but they hardly said a word to each other, so that I was left wondering if Roksana knew how to engage with her son at all.

'Oskar, it's Mummy.'

'Yes.'

Pause. 'Can you hear me?'

'Yes.'

Another pause. 'Are you all right?'

'Yes.'

More silence. 'I'm going to work now.'

'Yes.'

'Tell Mummy about school,' I prompted Oskar.

'I went to school,' he said uninspiringly.

'I know. I'll speak to you tomorrow. Be good. Bye.'

'Bye.'

The line went dead and Oskar passed the phone back to me. It was probably the shortest, saddest telephone conversation I'd ever heard between a mother and her son. There was so much they could have said. Clearly it wasn't only Roksana who'd had difficulty in talking; Oskar had been equally inhibited. However, as the parent, Roksana bore the responsibility for trying to engage with him, if she knew how, which I was doubting. Most parents, even those who have neglected or abused their children, can talk to them on the phone. In the past I'd often had to wind up a conversation or it would have gone on all night. I hoped that the next telephone contact – on Friday – would be better.

It was no different. Then, on Saturday evening, Oskar refused to speak to his mother at all and went to his bedroom. I explained to Roksana as tactfully as I could that Oskar didn't feel able to talk to her right now, and I didn't think it wise to insist.

'It's OK,' she said, far too accepting.

'We'll try again tomorrow. I'm sorry.'

'It's not your fault. He can be like that sometimes.' Most parents would have blamed me.

That night, I tried talking to Oskar about his mother and the phone calls, his life at home with her and whether there was anything worrying him, but I got no further than I had all the other times. Nods, shrugs and silence.

CHAPTER ELEVEN

NOT SAFE

On a positive note, during the weekend we managed to get Oskar playing some games. Weekends were easier, as we had more time, so he painted pictures, modelled in dough and built castles out of Lego, quietly and with the same self-contained approach he applied to most tasks. He hadn't asked for his toys from home, and I was hoping that his mother would bring them to contact at some point.

On Sunday we went to visit my mother – just Paula and Oskar came with me, as Adrian was seeing Kirsty and Lucy, Darren. Lucy had seen Darren on Friday and Saturday evening as well as at work during the week. In between, her phone frequently buzzed with text messages from him. I knew they were from him because she couldn't help but smile as she read each message and then immediately replied. I assumed everything was going well and hoped to meet him when she felt the time was right.

Oskar was a little more relaxed at Mum's on Sunday, possibly because it was his second visit. He managed to reply when she spoke to him and moved away from my side long enough to play with some of the toys in her toy box. But towards the end of the afternoon my brother popped in and I saw Oskar go on full alert. He jumped up from where he'd been sitting by the toy box and came to me. My brother was his usual chatty and friendly self, but Oskar shrank back whenever he spoke to him, and just nodded or shook his head in reply. I made the excuse that he hadn't been with us for long and was still shy, but it was the same reaction I'd seen in Oskar when he was around Adrian and Andrew – a wariness of men.

I was driving back from Mum's between five and six o'clock, so it was just after six when I telephoned Roksana. Oskar had promised me he would talk to her, but before I passed the phone to him I apologized to Roksana for phoning late and explained that we'd been to my mother's, which was an hour's drive away.

'It's OK,' Roksana said easily. 'I don't work on Sunday evenings. It's my one evening off.'

'You do work long hours,' I said.

'Yes. All day and most nights. I have to support Oskar and Luka.'

While I admired her work ethic, again I wondered what impact this had had on Oskar and how it would affect the social services' parenting assessment of her. In reality, she spent very little time with Oskar.

I'd already suggested to Oskar some things he could talk to his mother about – for example, what he'd been doing during the weekend – and it began well.

'I've been out for the day,' he said.

'So have I,' Roksana replied. 'I've been to work and now I'm on my way home.'

'I'm home now,' Oskar said, and was about to say more when she interrupted.

'No, you're not,' she said sharply. 'You're at your foster carer's house. Your home is with me. Don't forget that, Oskar.'

He looked crestfallen and after that all he would say was yes or no, and then, before long, goodbye. Their relationship appeared to be so fragile, it didn't take much for either of them to recoil, and I wondered how much good telephone contact was doing. However, it had been agreed between Roksana and Andrew, so until he told me otherwise I would continue to make the phone calls on the evenings they didn't see each other and hoped they improved.

When I collected Oskar from school on Monday afternoon I told him that Tamara, the Guardian, was visiting us and explained her role: a social worker who wanted to talk to him so she could tell the judge what was best for him long-term. Oskar was only six, but it was important he had some understanding of the court process and what it meant for him.

Tamara arrived promptly at four o'clock, shook my hand and smiled warmly at Oskar, who had come to the door with me. He managed a small hello.

Of average height and build, Tamara was in her fifties, smartly dressed in navy trousers, jacket and blouse. I knew from working with her before that she had a quiet, confident manner and was used to talking to children and eliciting a response. She accepted my offer of coffee and we sat in the living room, where she tried to engage Oskar in conversation but had no more success than Andrew had. She asked him about school and how that was going. 'Good. I like school,' he said. She asked him about seeing his mother and how that was. 'Yes,' he replied. She asked him if he liked living with me and he gave a small nod.

'Excellent,' Tamara replied, smiling at me.

She asked him if he had everything he needed from home. He didn't reply so I said, 'He has some of his clothes and I've bought what he needs. Roksana is going to let me have some more of his belongings, including some toys.'

'I'll remind her when I see her,' Tamara said, making a note. Then to Oskar, 'Do you understand why you are in care and living with Cathy?'

He nodded.

'Can you tell me?' He shook his head. 'Has your social worker told you?' He shrugged. 'It's because we want to make sure you are safe and well looked after.' He stared back at her.

'I'm seeing your mother next week,' Tamara continued. 'She has arranged to take an afternoon off work.' The fact that she'd mentioned Roksana taking time off work suggested it might have been an issue, but I knew that the Guardians only usually worked office hours, and it was expected that the parent(s) made time to see them. I hoped Roksana understood the importance of the Guardian's role.

Tamara then asked me how Oskar was settling in, about his routine and what he liked to do in his spare time as she made some notes. She gave me her business card listing her phone number and email address and said if Oskar or I had any questions I should contact her. She said she would see us at least once again before the final court hearing, which was set for October. She thanked me for my time and, having said goodbye to both of us, she left. Between now and October she would be gathering the information she needed to make a recommendation to the judge on whether Oskar could return to live with his mother.

It was now after five o'clock, so, setting the phone to speaker, I told Oskar it was time to call his mother. I said hello to Roksana and then passed the phone to him. 'How are you?' she asked.

'Another social worker was here,' he said.

'Who?' she asked anxiously. Oskar looked at me.

'It was the Guardian ad Litem,' I said into the speaker.

'What did she want?' she asked suspiciously. 'She's seeing me next week.'

'It's normal for the Guardian to see the child,' I said, which I was sure would have been explained to her.

'What did Oskar tell her?'

'That he liked school and understood why he was in care. Try not to worry.' I appreciated that parents with children in care must feel that a lot of meetings go on without them, which is true. I'm not the only one who would like to see more transparency in child-care proceedings. 'I'll let you and Oskar carry on chatting,' I said. 'Probably best not to quiz him about the Guardian's visit, though.'

'Have you been to school?' she asked him.

'Yes.'

'Have you got homework?'

'Yes.'

'Make sure you do it.'

'I will, I'm going to do it now,' he said. 'Bye.'

'Bye, I'll see you tomorrow.'

And that was that.

Of course I noted all this in my log as I was supposed to, while omitting my feeling that there was as much unsaid in these exchanges between Roksana and her son as there was said.

On Tuesday morning, notice of Oskar's review arrived in the post. It was set for the following Monday at 2 p.m. at Oskar's school. Children in care have regular reviews; the first takes place within four weeks of the child being placed or moving placement. The child's parent(s), social worker, teacher, foster carer, the foster carer's supervising social worker, and any other professionals or adults closely connected with the child are invited. Reviews are there to ensure that everything is being done to help the child, and that the care plan (drawn up by the social services) is up to date. They are chaired by an Independent Reviewing Officer (IRO), who also minutes the meeting. He is a qualified social worker with extra training but is unconnected with the social services. Very young children don't usually attend their reviews; older children are expected to.

I completed my review form that morning – it took almost an hour. It asked questions about Oskar's health, education, hobbies and interests, contact with family and friends, emotional well-being, and if the child's cultural and religious needs were being met. Oskar's form was a much shorter, child-friendly booklet designed to encourage the child to give their views on being in care. I'd help him complete it when we had the time and then post both forms to the reviewing officer, ready for the review on the following week.

That Tuesday afternoon, when Oskar and I arrived at the Family Centre, Roksana must have gone in just ahead of us. She was in reception signing the Visitors' Book.

'Hello,' I said. She turned.

At this point most parents and children would fall into each other's arms, but not Roksana and Oskar. Oskar dropped my hand but then looked at his mother carefully. Roksana declared, 'I'm so stressed! Luka is ill again and I can't afford to go back there now.'

'I am sorry to hear that,' I sympathized. 'What a worry for you.'

'It is!' she said. 'If it's not one thing, it's another!'

Oskar was looking anxious too, sharing his mother's worries.

'I'm sure Luka will be better soon,' I told him, feeling he needed some reassurance.

'I'm not,' Roksana declared. 'He keeps falling ill. As if I didn't have enough to cope with already – with Oskar being in care.' While I had every sympathy for her, I was concerned that Oskar could assume that being in care and all the worry it was causing his mother was his fault.

'Shall we go to the room?' I suggested, throwing Oskar a reassuring smile. I signed the Visitors' Book.

'You're in Green Room again,' the receptionist said, having heard our exchange. 'You can go through. The contact supervisor is there.'

I thanked her and we went through the double doors and began down the corridor towards the room.

'I know where it is,' Roksana said curtly to me. 'You don't have to come with us.'

'I'm supposed to see you into the room,' I replied.

'Don't they trust me?'

'It's policy,' I said diplomatically. But of course, had Roksana wanted to threaten Oskar not to tell, she could have done so in the short distance from reception to the room. There have been instances of a parent intimidating their child when they've gone to the toilet or to the kitchen for a glass of water. If the contact supervisor was doing her job properly, she wouldn't let Roksana or Oskar out of her sight for a second.

Once in Green Room I said goodbye and have a nice time, then left. As contact was only an hour it wasn't worth me going home. The weather was fine, so I went for a walk and then returned to collect Oskar at five o'clock. I knocked on the door and went in. It was very quiet and the room was tidy, so any games they'd been playing with had already been packed away. My first impression was that Roksana was a little less stressed. 'Everything OK?' I asked her, just being friendly.

'Yes. I've been on the phone to my sister and Luka has stopped being sick,' she said. 'It seems it was just a stomach upset. He's prone to getting them.'

'That's a relief,' I said. But I looked at Oskar sitting passively on the sofa and wondered how much of the hour's contact had been dedicated to him and how much to Luka. I appreciated what a worry it must be for Roksana, but I felt sorry for Oskar, who seemed to take second place – to his mother's work and Luka.

It's usual for the foster carer to leave the Family Centre with the child first to avoid any emotional or difficult situations developing outside, so I said goodbye to Roksana and that we'd phone her tomorrow.

'Goodbye,' Oskar said, standing, and he came straight to me.

'Are you going to give your mother a kiss goodbye?' I asked him.

Roksana had stood and was now checking her phone. Oskar dutifully returned to her. Not taking her eyes from her phone, she threw a half-hearted kiss in the direction of his head. No hug, no proper kiss goodbye. As he returned to me, I saw the look of disappointment on his face and I wished Roksana could have seen it too. Children thrive on attention and praise, and wither from emotional neglect.

'Good boy,' I said, smiling at him, and he took my hand.

Outside, I asked him if he'd had a nice time and he said, 'Yes,' although his voice was flat. I then asked him if he would like to invite a friend from school home for tea one afternoon, and he shrugged gloomily. 'Think about it,' I said. But I was beginning to wonder if Oskar was depressed. It was relatively unusual for a child of his age to be depressed, but it was something I would raise with his social worker. Some children are referred to CAMHS (Child and Adolescent Mental Health Services) for therapy when they come into care.

On Wednesday the phone call to Roksana was no better or worse than the previous ones. It was very short and uninspiring, and Oskar responded to his mother's questions with 'Yes', 'No' or a shrug, which of course she couldn't see. I prompted him with some topics he could talk to her about, but with the phone on speaker Roksana could hear me and said, 'It's OK if he doesn't want to talk,' and she said goodbye.

After dinner that evening I took out Oskar's review form and explained to him what the review was all about, then we sat at the table in the kitchen-diner to complete it. He could read some of the questions and his writing was about average for a six-year-old. Some of the questions had a choice of emojis and didn't require a written answer. To begin with his responses were pretty much what I would have expected of him.

How do you feel most of the time? He circled the emoji with a sad face.

Would you like to know more about your past? 'Don't mind,' he wrote.

Who is your social worker? 'Andrew.'

Would you like to see more of them? 'No.'

Who are your friends? Would you like to see more of them? 'Don't mind.'

If you have any problems, who do you talk to? 'Miss Jordan.'

'I hope you can talk to me too,' I reminded Oskar, and he nodded.

Do you have any questions about what is going to happen in the future? Most children would put: 'When can I go home?' But to my astonishment Oskar wrote: 'Can I stay with Cathy?'

I turned and looked at him carefully. 'Do you want to stay with me?' I asked. 'Or is it you think that's what I want to hear?'

'No, it's true,' he said in a tiny voice.

'Why?'

He didn't reply but read the next question: *Is there anything you would like to add?*

He paused thoughtfully and then wrote: 'I don't want to go home.'

'Can you write why you don't want to go home?' I asked. It's often easier to write something painful than to say it.

He paused again and then wrote: 'It's not safe.'

'Why isn't it safe?' I asked. 'Write it down.'

'No, I can't tell you,' he whispered, and concentrated on the next question.

CHAPTER TWELVE

MR NOWAK

I was reeling from the shock of Oskar's disclosure – that he'd admitted he didn't feel safe at home – as he quietly signed his review form. I'd looked after children before who'd been able to write down something bad that had happened to them when they hadn't been able to say it, but I'd never had a child actually disclose on their review form. I'd always found the questions rather bland, but clearly they had allowed Oskar to say how he was feeling when he hadn't been able to tell me or Andrew. I reassured him he was safe with me, but I couldn't make promises about where he would live long-term, as that was for the judge to decide in October. I also said that I'd need to tell Andrew what he'd told me about not feeling safe at home, which Oskar accepted with a small nod. Was his comment referring solely to the bruise he'd arrived with on his face from being slapped? I doubted it. In my experience children put up with a lot worse than a slap and still want to return home.

Once Oskar was in bed that evening I wrote up my log notes, including exactly what he'd said, and also sent an email to his social worker updating him. I put the review forms in the envelope provided, ready to post the following day. Not only Andrew, but everyone present at the review would appreciate the significance of Oskar's disclosure, and I wondered what his mother would have to say. The IRO would refer to Oskar's review form as part of the review, and often they read it out, with the child's permission.

That night Oskar had a nightmare and I found him buried deep under his duvet, hot, trembling and with his eyes screwed tightly shut. He was trying to fight off something or someone, and it took me a while to bring him out of it. I sat with him until he was in a peaceful sleep again and returned to my bed, although it was a long time before I fell asleep. Foster carers worry about the child they look after as much, if not more, than they do their own children, for they've already suffered a lot.

On Thursday, Roksana was fifteen minutes late for contact and rushed into the room, stressed. 'My last lady had an accident just as I was about to leave,' she said. 'So I had to stop and change her again.'

'You're a carer as well as a cleaner?' I asked.

'Yes, I clean offices early morning and evening, and I work as an agency carer during the day.' She sighed.

Not wanting to impinge on her time with Oskar, I said goodbye to them both and left. They wouldn't be allowed extra time to make up for Roksana being late, as it's considered the responsibly of the parent to make sure they attend each contact session punctually. While one unavoidable lateness wouldn't count against her, it would if it became a regular occurrence. There are rules about contact at the Family Centre, which the parent is made aware of; for example, if they're half an hour late without phoning to say they're on their way, the session is cancelled and the carer takes the child home. While it's disappointing for all concerned, it's not as upsetting for the child as having to wait indefinitely for a parent who may not arrive at all. If a parent keeps failing to arrive then contact is often suspended. Harsh though this may seem, it is to protect the child from the pain of further let-downs and rejection – which their lives have often been full of.

When I collected Oskar at the end of contact the room was quiet and tidy as usual, and, as before, mother and son separated easily – too easily for my liking. I hoped I would get some more feedback about contact from Andrew before long.

On Saturday morning I took Oskar for dental and optician check-ups as the foster carer is expected to do. This is in addition to the medical the social worker arranges. His teeth and eyesight were fine, and afterwards I took him to an activity centre. He'd never been to one before, and after some initial reluctance on his part he played and enjoyed himself for an hour or so. On Sunday we didn't visit my mother as she was going to my brother's for dinner. It was a lovely, warm May morning and I suggested to Oskar that we take a football to the park. Adrian said he could come, as he wasn't seeing Kirsty. Most lads I'd fostered would have been delighted to have Adrian with us, as many of them, like Oskar, had a single-parent mother so had often lacked a good male role model. Indeed, it was something I'd been concerned about after my husband had left me when my children had been young. But my dear father had stepped into that role and done a great job.

Sadly, Oskar showed the same wariness towards Adrian as he had done previously and tucked himself into my side as we walked to the park, as far away from Adrian as possible. Thankfully Adrian was easy-going and used to a range of behaviours from the children we fostered, so he didn't take it personally. Indeed, he might not even have noticed.

Once in the park we went over to the playing-field area and Adrian began kicking the ball about with the intention of encouraging Oskar to join in. Others were playing in small family groups and with friends. Oskar watched Adrian until I joined in and kicked the ball to Oskar and then he returned it to me and finally Adrian. After that, the three of us kicked the ball between us for half an hour or so and Oskar seemed to enjoy himself. We then went to the area where the children's apparatus was, and while Oskar went on the swings and roundabout, Adrian and I talked – to begin with about his job as a trainee accountant. We didn't get much time to talk just the two of us, so I made the most of it.

'How are you and Kirsty?' I asked nonchalantly when he'd finished telling me about work.

'Fine, Mum.'

'Good. She's lovely. You know I like her a lot.'

He smiled indulgently. 'Yes, and now I have a permanent job I can save up more.'

'Very good. What for?'

'A deposit on a flat.'

'With Kirsty?'

'Yes, of course, Mum.'

'That's nice.'

I'd thought as much, but I find, when it comes to romance and one's children, it's best not to take things for granted. Adrian and Kirsty had been dating steadily since college and I hoped they would make a future together, although I was in no rush for him to leave.

We returned home and I cooked Sunday lunch, after which Lucy disappeared off to see Darren. 'Don't be too late, you've got work tomorrow,' I reminded her. She'd been out with him until late on Friday and Saturday.

'I won't!' she called, and the front door closed behind her.

When Oskar and I telephoned his mother that evening it was their usual short exchange, and when they'd finished I added, 'See you tomorrow at the review, Roksana.'

'No, I can't go,' she said. 'I've left Andrew a message. I have to work.'

'Oh dear, that's a pity. Can't you swap shifts?'

'It's impossible. I've told Andrew.'

'OK. We'll phone as usual in the evening then.' We said goodbye.

I hoped Roksana appreciated the importance of attending her child's review. Going would have shown a level of commitment and also given her the chance to see Oskar, but it wasn't for me to tell her.

On Monday morning, as I drove to school, I reminded Oskar about his review that afternoon. I'd already told him what to expect. As we waited for school to start Miss Jordan came into the playground, asked us if we'd had a good weekend and then said she'd be attending the review but wasn't sure of the format. I told her much the same as I'd told Oskar.

'It's nothing to worry about,' I added, for she looked quite nervous.

'How long do you think I should speak for?' she asked.

'About five or ten minutes. Just say how Oskar is doing academically and socially – mixing with his peers.'

'Should I bring him to the review with me?'

'No, see what the chairperson suggests. They may want him there at the beginning or just towards the end. Someone can always leave the review to fetch him from the classroom if necessary.'

'Thank you,' she said, still a little nervous. 'I'll see you later then.'

'You'll be fine. Don't worry.'

'Don't worry, Miss,' Oskar said cutely, and we both smiled. I could appreciate how daunting it must seem to her. I remembered how I used to feel when I had first begun to attend reviews and other meetings connected with fostering. Even now, I felt a little anxious just before a meeting, as they are quite formal.

I hadn't been home long when Andrew telephoned, having read the email I'd sent him on Friday evening. He wanted an update prior to the review. I went over what Oskar had said about wanting to stay with me as he didn't feel safe at home when he'd completed his review form. 'Has he said any more?'

'No, although he had another nightmare on Friday night.'

'I've made a referral to CAMHS, but there is a waiting list.'

At 12.30 I made myself a sandwich lunch, then I changed into a smart outfit and with my notes in my shoulder bag I drove to Oskar's school. I arrived ten minutes before the review was due to begin. Andrew was in reception signing the Visitors' Book. He said hello and passed the pen to me. 'I'm just waiting to hear which room we are in,' he said.

At that moment Elaine Summer, the Head Teacher, appeared through a set of double doors to our right and said good afternoon.

'The Independent Reviewing Officer has just arrived and I've shown him into our meeting room,' she said. 'This way.'

As Andrew and I followed her along the corridor she said she would stay for at least part of the review. It wasn't essential she was present, as Miss Jordan was attending. We went up a small flight of stairs and into a carpeted room where a large table stood in the centre with chairs around it. 'This used to be a classroom,' Elaine Summer explained. 'But numbers on our roll fell so we use it for meetings now.' Miss Jordan was already sitting at the table, as was a man I took to be the IRO. Andrew and I said hello to them and I threw Miss Jordan a reassuring smile and sat down. The IRO had his laptop open and was quietly studying the screen. I took out my notes and set them on the table in front of me, while Andrew took a folder from his briefcase.

After a few minutes the door opened and Edith, my SSW, came in. 'I am in the right room then,' she said and sat beside me.

'Are we expecting anyone else?' the IRO asked Andrew. 'I've received an apology for absence from the Guardian ad Litem. Is Oskar's mother attending? It's two o'clock.'

'No, she sends her apologies. She has to work.'

'She couldn't get the time off?' he asked.

'Apparently not,' Andrew replied. 'She's had a lot of time off in the last month.'

'Would it be helpful if we offered a different time for the next review?' the IRO asked. 'It is important she feels able to attend if she wishes to.'

'I'll speak to her again, but Roksana works very long hours,' Andrew replied, and made a note.

'So we're all here?' the IRO checked.

'Yes,' Andrew said.

'Shall I fetch Oskar now?' Miss Jordan asked nervously.

The IRO looked at Andrew. 'I suggest we hear from

the adults present first and then bring Oskar in towards the end.'

'That's fine with me,' Andrew confirmed.

'Let's begin with the introductions,' the IRO said. 'This is the first review for Oskar. My name is Graham Hitchens, Independent Reviewing Officer.' We then went round the table stating our names and role as the IRO typed, ending with Elaine Summer, Head Teacher. 'And Oskar is in care under an Interim Care Order?' he confirmed with Andrew.

'Yes.'

The IRO finished typing and looked at me. 'Thank you for returning the review forms.' I was now expecting him to ask me to give my report first. It's usual for the foster carer to go first, as they have the most up-to-date information on the child. But before he could get any further, a knock sounded on the door. We all looked over. The door opened and the school secretary took a step in. 'One of Oskar's uncles, Mr Nowak, is in reception,' she said. 'He says he is here to attend the review in place of Roksana, as she is at work.'

This was highly unusual and we looked at the IRO.

'Was he invited?' the IRO asked Andrew.

'No, it's the first I've heard of it.'

'I don't think it's appropriate then,' he said.

'He's been very insistent,' the secretary said. 'He says he's brought some more of Oskar's clothes and toys, as Roksana can't take them on the bus.'

'Mr Nowak is the one who has been bringing Oskar to school and collecting him the most,' the Head added.

'I met him here the afternoon Oskar was brought into care,' Andrew said. 'But my understanding is that he is a family friend and not a relative.'

The IRO looked thoughtful. While it was unusual for someone to arrive at a review uninvited, it wasn't unheard of. When it had happened to me it had been an angry parent and her partner who had turned up, wanting to confront and disrupt the review. There was good reason why they'd been stopped from attending their child's reviews, as their behaviour had been very threatening in the past. The police were called to escort them from the premises, but Mr Nowak didn't have a track record of threatening behaviour as far as I knew.

'What shall I tell him?' the secretary asked, still half in and half out of the door. 'He says he has something important to say.'

'I think it might be prudent if we listened to him as long as he understands he won't be staying for the whole meeting,' the IRO suggested. Andrew agreed.

'Perhaps you'd like to come and tell him?' the secretary said.

Andrew stood, so too did the IRO. 'I'll come with you,' he said.

'Do you want me there?' the Head asked.

'No, we'll speak to him,' the IRO replied.

The atmosphere was now rather tense and Miss Jordan was looking worried again. Her first review and it wasn't going to plan – far from it.

'He definitely wasn't one of the men waiting in the car?' I asked the Head.

'No. I'd have recognized Mr Nowak,' she replied.

'What's all this about?' Edith asked. I had told her about the two men waiting outside the school, but clearly she'd forgotten. I briefly explained, and she made a note.

'You haven't seen them since I spoke to them?' the Head asked me.

'No, and I've checked with Oskar a few times and he hasn't either.'

We sat in silence as we waited; the only sound came from the old-fashioned wall clock as it ticked off the minutes. At 2.15 footsteps could be heard approaching in the corridor outside and the door opened. The IRO came in first, followed by Andrew and Mr Nowak. My stomach clenched to a tight ball. I recognized Mr Nowak. True, he wasn't one of the men in the car, but I had seen him a few times on the opposite side of the road to the school when I'd collected Oskar. He was tall and distinguished-looking, with quite sharp features, so easily recognizable. Whether Oskar had seen him I didn't know; he certainly hadn't said anything to me.

'Do sit down,' the IRO said as he and Andrew returned to their seats.

'No, thank you. I stand,' Mr Nowak replied in broken English. 'I have something to say and then I go.' All eyes were on him and he met my gaze. In that moment I knew he realized I'd recognized him. 'I left Oskar's bag downstairs,' he said, and I nodded.

'The secretary has it in her office,' Andrew told me.

'Thank you,' I said quietly. I wasn't sure at what point I should say I recognized him.

He remained standing as he spoke and addressed us all. I guessed he'd rehearsed what he had to say: 'The boy's mother works hard. She has a sick son. It's bad she has to worry about Oskar. It is wrong he has been taken away. I know her for many years. She is a good mother but has a hard life. You must give her son back to her. That is what I came to say.'

While this appeared commendable and his sentiment well meant, I was concerned as to why he had been waiting outside the school, and it was clear he had little understanding of the function of a review.

'Thank you, Mr Nowak,' the IRO said, glancing up from his laptop as he paused from typing. 'I have noted your comments. I'm afraid reviews like this cannot change the decision of the court. Oskar will need to remain in foster care until the judge hears all the evidence and makes a decision on where he will live permanently.'

'He should live with his mother,' Mr Nowak replied more sharply.

'That will be for the judge to decide,' the IRO said. 'Has Roksana seen a solicitor?'

Mr Nowak looked puzzled and I guessed it was the term solicitor he didn't understand.

'Yes,' Andrew said. Then to Mr Nowak: 'Roksana saw a lawyer for legal advice.'

'He told her it take months before court,' Mr Nowak said. 'October. The boy has to go home now.'

'I'm afraid that's not possible,' the IRO said firmly as the rest of us remained quiet. 'I suggest Roksana talks to her lawyer if she has concerns. Is there anything else you wish to say?'

'It's bad you have her son,' he said quite vehemently.

'I've noted your comments,' the IRO said. 'Is that everything?'

While this had been going on, I'd become increasingly convinced that I should say something about him being outside the school. Certainly, I would tell Andrew after the meeting, but then I found myself saying: 'Mr Nowak, I've seen you waiting outside the school when I've collected Oskar.'

Everyone looked at me and then at Mr Nowak, their expressions serious. 'I tell his mother he is OK,' he replied.

'That is why I look. She worries but has to work, so she asks me.'

The Head and Miss Jordan were clearly surprised by his admission and unaware he had been outside the school.

'I think it's better if you don't wait outside the school any more,' the IRO said firmly. 'It could worry and unsettle Oskar. If Roksana wants to know about her son, she can ask her social worker, Andrew, and she sees Oskar at contact.'

'It is not right!' Mr Nowak said. 'The boy should be home with his mother!' Turning, he headed for the door.

'I'll see you out,' the Head said, standing, and quickly followed him.

As the door closed, I wasn't the only one who breathed a sigh of relief, and I felt sorry for Miss Jordan, who had experienced such a disruptive start to her first review.

CHAPTER THIRTEEN

REVIEW

While we waited for the Head Teacher to return to the review, the IRO asked me how often I had seen Mr Nowak outside the school. I said I couldn't be sure, but I thought three or four times, and that Oskar had never mentioned it. Miss Jordan said Oskar hadn't told her either and drew the conclusion that Mr Nowak's presence wasn't therefore worrying Oskar.

'Or it might be that he felt he couldn't tell us,' I said. 'I have the feeling there's a lot Oskar should be telling us but isn't.'

She gave a slow, thoughtful nod. 'He is very quiet in school. He always has been.'

'I'll speak to his mother again,' Andrew said, 'and make sure she understands she can have more contact if she wishes, but that it isn't appropriate for her to send anyone to wait outside the school.'

The IRO agreed that was advisable.

It was now 2.30 and the review hadn't properly started. Usually they last for about an hour, but clearly we were going to overrun. Five minutes later the Head returned and the IRO asked her if Mr Nowak had left.

'Yes, he wasn't any trouble,' she said, returning to her seat. 'I think he's sincere. We've had a chat and he has promised he won't hang around outside the school again, although of course that remains to be seen. I've had this problem before with children in care and those whose parents are separating. The estranged parent knows where the school is and what time the child comes out, so they wait to catch a glimpse of them. It's sad, really.' She had said similar to me before about the two men in the car.

'But it's still unsettling for the child,' Edith said, and I agreed.

The IRO now asked me to give my report and I glanced at my notes. I always like to start with the positives. 'Oskar is a lovely child, kind, sensitive and caring,' I said as the IRO typed. 'He likes school and learning and has no behavioural problems, either at home or at school. I've suggested he might like to invite a friend home to play and he's thinking about it.' I paused to allow the IRO time to catch up.

'Oskar is in good health,' I continued. 'I took him for his medical, and also dental and opticians check-ups. He doesn't need glasses and his teeth are in good condition. However, he appears quite anxious and withdrawn most of the time and I understand Andrew has made a referral to CAMHS.' I paused again and glanced at my notes.

'Oskar sees his mother at the Family Centre for an hour twice a week and has phone contact on the other nights. Oskar is fine about attending and isn't upset afterwards.'

'Is he excited at the prospect of seeing his mother?' the IRO asked.

'Not really excited. I would say more accepting – he seems to accept whatever comes his way.'

'That's worrying,' the IRO said as he typed.

'It is,' I agreed.

'And the phone contact? How is that?' he asked.

'They both seem to find it quite difficult. Their conversations are very short, no more than a couple of minutes, and they don't really say much. I suppose it could be because I am listening. Andrew asked me to monitor the phone contact.'

The IRO nodded and typed.

'Oskar has been having nightmares,' I continued. 'Although he won't talk about them afterwards, he seems to be fighting someone off and telling them to leave him alone. He also appears to be wary around adult men. I've noticed it with my son, my brother and also when Andrew visited him.' Andrew nodded.

'Has this been noticed in school?' the IRO asked the Head.

'We don't have any male teachers here, only a male teaching assistant and he's not in Oskar's class. We have a male caretaker, but there's no reason for Oskar to come into contact with him.'

The IRO looked to me to continue.

'Oskar is very anxious about undressing in front of anyone. I give him privacy when he has a bath and gets ready for bed. In my experience most children his age aren't self-conscious. He was very worried about being examined at his medical. I don't know if the paediatrician mentioned it in her report.'

'Yes, she did,' Andrew confirmed.

'How is he about changing for PE?' the Head asked Miss Jordan.

She hesitated and then said, 'I hadn't really thought about it until now, but Oskar doesn't change with the other children. He always says he has to use the toilet and when he comes out he's changed. I probably should have reported it, but I didn't think anything of it.' She looked worried and I threw her a reassuring smile.

'Has there been any suggestion that Oskar has been sexually abused?' the IRO asked Andrew.

'No, but of course it is possible.'

'I have the feeling Oskar has secrets that he's too scared to tell,' I now said, addressing the IRO. 'He wrote on his review form that he wanted to stay with me, as it wasn't safe at home.'

'Really?' Miss Jordan gasped.

'I saw that,' the IRO said.

'I asked Oskar if he could tell me why he didn't feel safe at home, but he couldn't. It might come out in time or in therapy, but I understand there is a long waiting list for CAMHS.'

'There is,' Andrew confirmed. 'Oskar's case isn't classified as urgent.'

The IRO finished typing and looked up. 'Thank you, Cathy. Is there anything else you want to add?'

'No, I don't think so.'

'And Oskar can stay with you for as long as necessary?' It was a standard question at a review.

'Yes.'

'Thank you. Would you like to give your report next?' the IRO asked Andrew. All eyes turned to him.

Andrew began by confirming the date Oskar had been brought into care, the reasons and the type of court order granted. 'Roksana was abroad at the time because her other son, Luka, was ill,' he said. 'Luka lives with her sister. Since Roksana returned I have met with her three times, once at her home address.'

'Is Luka the only other sibling?' the IRO asked.

'Yes,' Andrew confirmed, and continued his report. 'While Roksana was abroad she left Oskar in the care of various adults in the house where she lives. Oskar refers to them as aunts and uncles, but none of them are related to him. Initially Roksana was adamant that Oskar was always clean, well fed and being looked after, but she has since admitted that because of the long hours she works she is rarely at home and relies heavily on the others in the house. In reality, she has very little input into Oskar's daily care and says he is self-sufficient.'

'Is Roksana there in the morning to make Oskar breakfast and take him to school?' the IRO asked.

'No. One of her jobs is as an office cleaner with a start time of six in the morning.'

'And the evening?' the IRO asked.

'She's rarely home before ten.'

I saw Elaine Summer frown. 'We've only seen her at the school once,' she said. 'When she first registered Oskar.'

'That's feasible,' Andrew said. 'Others in the house have been bringing Oskar and collecting him, and making him meals and so forth. At any one time there are between twelve and sixteen adults living in the house and they share child-care.'

'Are there other children living there now?' the IRO asked.

'Not at present, and we're trying to trace the children who have been living there. Some have returned abroad to live, but others have moved within the UK. I've had to tell Roksana that the house, as it is, isn't suitable for children.'

'No, indeed,' the Head agreed.

'I've seen similar multiple-occupancy houses,' Andrew continued, 'and standards vary. They are often used by students and immigrant workers on zero-hours contracts, as the rents are low. Roksana's house was reasonably clean when I visited, but it is badly overcrowded and I've alerted the council, who will be assessing it.'

'So just to clarify,' the IRO said. 'No one person in the house was responsible for Oskar when his mother was away or at work?'

'That's correct,' Andrew said.

'And those living in the house are all well known to her?'

'No. A couple are friends she has known for a few years, but most of the others she doesn't know well. Some hadn't been there for long.'

The IRO nodded, the Head frowned again and Andrew continued. 'Initially Roksana was adamant no one in the house would harm Oskar and that he must have sustained the bruise on his face by falling over. She has now admitted that one of the men who was living in the house could have hit Oskar in anger. He was only there a few months but had a drink problem and a bad temper. She said one of the women told her that while she was away Oskar was cheeky to him, so he slapped him, hard.'

'Cheeky!' I exclaimed in disbelief. 'I can't imagine Oskar being cheeky to anyone!'

'Neither can I,' Miss Jordan added.

'Where did Oskar sleep at home?' the IRO asked Andrew.

'In a sleeping bag, on a mattress on the floor. All those living there have a sleeping bag. Four of the rooms have mattresses covering the floors, one of the rooms is used as a sitting room and they share the kitchen and bathroom. There is also a shower cubicle on each floor, but Roksana said only one works.'

'Who sleeps in the same room as Oskar?' the IRO asked, frowning.

'Other women he calls aunts.'

'Always women? No men?' he asked.

'Not according to Roksana. The single men have their own bedroom, and the couples have the two other bedrooms.'

'So presumably the mother thought these arrangements were acceptable?' the IRO asked.

Elaine Summer threw me a knowing look and I guessed we were thinking the same: living in an overcrowded house with strangers and so little parenting, Oskar was highly vulnerable – anything might have happened to him.

'Yes,' Andrew replied. 'Roksana said in her country most families have very basic accommodation and many share, as it's the only way to earn enough money to survive. I have had to make it clear to her that we don't consider it appropriate for a child to live like that here.'

Andrew glanced at his notes again. 'Contact,' he said, moving on. 'It is twice a week for an hour at the Family Centre. I was present at the first contact and I've read the supervisor's notes for the others. Roksana has attended each session but was late for one. The contact supervisor noted that Roksana and Oskar appear to struggle to interact and play together. Roksana is often anxious and constantly checks her phone. Oskar is very quiet and usually amuses himself by looking at books. A few times Roksana tried to tell him that his aunts and uncles in the house were good people and missed him and wanted him home. Oskar looked very worried and the supervisor intervened and told Roksana it was making Oskar anxious and shouldn't be discussed. I will attend contact again in a month.'

'Thank you,' the IRO said. 'And the care plan is the same?' It was a standard question.

'That's right,' Andrew said. 'Oskar will remain in care. There are no plans to return him home.'

'Miss Jordan, would you like to go next?' the IRO said.

She flushed up as she began. 'I have printed copies of Oskar's PEP,' she said. 'Shall I hand them out?'

'Yes, please,' the IRO said.

PEP stands for Personal Education Plan and it is a document drawn up to help a child in care reach their full potential. It shows where the child is now in their learning and sets out targets and actions for the coming term. It forms part of the care plan. As I looked at Oskar's PEP it was clear that academically he was doing well but he needed to participate more in class. Miss Jordan gave us a moment to read the PEP and then began her report.

'Oskar is a pleasant and studious member of my class. He applies himself well to tasks and gets on with his work without any fuss. He is working above average in all the core subjects, English, maths and science. However, he is very quiet and needs a lot of encouragement to participate in group discussion. Prior to him coming into care, I had very little to do with his care-givers, but now I see Cathy regularly in the playground. Oskar disclosed to me about how he got the bruise, but he hasn't given me any more details since. I would pass it on to Elaine Summer and Cathy if he did. When Oskar was first taken from his mother I was very worried for him, but now I can see how much he has improved. He arrives at school on time and is clean. I just wish he was happier. That's it, really.' She sat back, relieved.

'Thank you,' the IRO said. 'Why do you think Oskar is unhappy?'

'I don't know, perhaps because of what has happened to him. He looks sad most of the time, but he won't tell me why.'

'I understand,' the IRO said as he typed, then he looked at Elaine Summer: 'Would you like to add anything?'

'Yes, but it's more about procedure than about Oskar specifically. Miss Jordan has covered that. We reported our concerns that Oskar was being neglected when he first began attending this school at the start of the year, then again a month later when I spoke to a social worker – not Andrew – but nothing happened until Oskar came to school with a bruise while his mother was away. Why the delay?'

'I am sorry,' Andrew said, meeting her gaze. 'There seems to have been a breakdown in communication. I'll pass on what you've said.' He made a note.

So often a member of staff is the first to notice signs of neglect or abuse in a child they teach, as they see them most days. There are reporting strategies in place to make sure these concerns are looked into, but clearly something had gone wrong here.

'Thank you,' the IRO said to the Head, and he turned to Edith, my SSW. 'Would you like to add anything? Then we'll hear from Oskar.'

Edith said, as she usually did, that her role was to supervise, support and monitor my fostering. 'I visit her every month, when we discuss the child in placement,' she continued. 'Cathy is an experienced foster carer and I am satisfied Oskar is receiving a good standard of care.'

'Thank you,' the IRO said. 'Any complaints from anyone?' It was another standard question and those present either shook their head or said no.

'Would you like to fetch Oskar now?' the IRO asked Miss Jordan. She stood, as did the Head. 'School ends soon,' Elaine Summer said. 'I like to be in the playground as the children leave. Miss Jordan can tell me what I miss. Can you send the school a copy of the minutes, please?'

'Yes,' the IRO confirmed. It was usual for minutes of the

review to be circulated to all those who had been invited, whether they had attended or not. I wondered what Roksana would make of what had been said.

Both teachers left the room, and as the rest of us waited the bell sounded for the end of school. Five minutes later Miss Jordan returned with Oskar by her side. He was now looking even more worried and sad than usual. It must have been daunting for him to suddenly have to face us adults in the formal setting of the meeting room.

'Hello, love,' I said. 'Come and sit down.'

Oskar came over, head slightly bowed, and sat in the chair beside me. He looked so small in front of the large table.

'Welcome to your review,' the IRO said gently with a smile.

Oskar looked up cautiously.

'It's nothing to worry about,' I told him. Miss Jordan was smiling encouragingly at him too.

'How are you doing, Oskar?' the IRO asked.

'OK,' Oskar said quietly.

'Thank you for coming to your review. This is about you, so I'd like to ask you some questions to hear your views. Is that all right?' He gave a small nod.

'Do you like school?'

'Yes,' Oskar replied in the same small voice.

'Do you like living with Cathy?'

'Yes.'

'That's good. Thank you for completing your review form.' The IRO had it open in front of him and turned the pages. Oskar was watching him. 'You've put that you feel sad most of the time. Can you tell us why?'

Oskar shook his head.

'Shall I read out what you have put in your form?'

'No,' Oskar said quietly.

'That's all right.' The IRO wasn't taking notes but concentrating on Oskar. So were the rest of us.

'Do you have everything you need at Cathy's?' the IRO asked.

'Yes.'

'There are some more of your belongings in reception and Cathy will take them home with you. Is there anything else you want from home?'

'No,' he said. Then, taking a deep breath, he found the courage to say, 'I don't want to go home.'

Miss Jordan caught my gaze.

'I know you don't,' the IRO said encouragingly. 'You wrote that on your form, and that you didn't feel safe at home. Can you tell us why?'

Oskar thought for a moment and then shook his head.

'Do you know who you can tell if you want to?' he asked. Oskar nodded, but the IRO said, 'Your social worker, Andrew; your foster carer, Cathy; your teacher, Miss Jordan, or another adult you trust.'

Oskar gave another small nod. While he clearly wasn't going to add anything more to what he'd put on his review form, the fact that he had been able to speak out suggested we were slowly inching closer to the point where he could tell someone. It was important he did, for, like other children I'd fostered, he clearly carried a huge burden, which would scar his life until he shared it.

CHAPTER FOURTEEN

DISTRAUGHT

On our way out of the school I collected the bag Mr Nowak had left with the school secretary. Oskar tucked his hand into mine and we crossed the playground and headed towards my car. As we walked I praised him and said he'd done well to attend his review. He didn't reply. I then asked him, 'Have you ever seen your Uncle Nowak waiting outside the school?'

'Yes,' he replied easily.

'Why didn't you tell me, love?'

'He's nice. I don't mind him here.'

I unlocked the car. 'Have you ever seen anyone else you know, apart from him, waiting outside the school? Those two men in the black car?'

'No. I don't see them any more.'

'All right. You must tell me if you do.'

'I just see Uncle Nowak and he tells Mummy I'm OK,' Oskar said, clambering into the back seat.

'How do you know that?' I asked.

'Mummy told me at contact,' he said and fastened his seatbelt.

I let the matter drop and closed his car door. But why on earth had no one thought to tell me what Roksana had told

Oskar during contact? Foster carers don't receive a copy of the contact supervisor's reports, but here was a good example of why we should. Information sharing has improved since I first began fostering, but it still has a long way to go.

Once home, I took the bag of Oskar's belongings up to his room to sort through later and then set about making dinner. Oskar, never far from my side, sat at the table in the kitchen-diner looking at some books as I worked. He would go to Lucy and Paula sometimes, but never Adrian. I assumed the reason he liked to keep me in sight was because I was his main care-giver.

After we'd had dinner and Oskar had telephoned his mother (it was their usual short exchange), I suggested to him that we go upstairs and unpack his bag. 'It will be nice for you to have some more of your toys from home,' I said.

He didn't reply but, always compliant, came with me. He wasn't excited at the prospect of being reunited with his toys as most children would have been.

'What you don't want I can put away,' I said. Ultimately these items would be returned to his mother, whether Oskar went home or not, as legally they were hers.

Oskar followed me into his bedroom, where I unzipped the laundry-style bag and began taking out his clothes, which were neatly packed at the top. Oskar stood, watching me. I laid the clothes in little piles on his bed. These clothes were much newer than the ones that had previously been sent from home while Roksana had been away. I remembered her telling me that the friend who'd packed Oskar's belongings hadn't included his good clothes that she'd worked so hard to afford.

'These are nice,' I said, holding up a pair of jogging bottoms. 'You'll be able to wear them.' Oskar wasn't interested, but I wouldn't have expected a six-year-old to show much interest in clothes. He'd be more interested in the toys I had now uncovered at the bottom of the bag. I started taking them out and setting them on the floor. 'Wow!' I said. 'A remote-controlled car. A talking, walking robot. *Star Wars* models. And your very own tablet!' They were all brand new and two were still in their boxes.

'You'll have fun playing with these,' I said, glancing at him. But he was backing away, staring at them, horrified.

'Whatever is the matter?' I asked.

'I don't want them,' he said, his face crumpling.

'Because they remind you of home?'

'No. They hurt me.'

'The toys hurt you?' I looked at them, puzzled. I couldn't see how they might be dangerous. They were for children his age, including the tablet, and didn't have any sharp edges.

'Throw them away!' he cried, bursting into tears. Then he wet himself.

I immediately went to him.

'I'm sorry,' he wept.

'It's all right. Don't upset yourself.' I took his hand. 'All children have accidents. Let's get you into the bath.'

'Shall I clear it up?' he asked in a small voice.

'No, of course not. I'll do that. Do you need to go to the toilet now?'

'No,' he mumbled through his tears.

'Come on, it's OK. Don't worry,' I reassured him and led him towards the bathroom.

As we passed Paula's bedroom I knocked on her door. 'Could you give me a hand, please?'

She must have heard Oskar crying, for she opened her door straight away, looking concerned. 'Can you stay with

Oskar, please, and start running his bath while I pop downstairs and get a bucket?' It was obvious he'd wet himself as the front of his trousers were wet.

Paula can sometimes be a bit squeamish about these matters, unlike Lucy, who is used to dealing with children having accidents at the nursery, but Lucy was out with Darren. Paula stepped up to the mark and, taking Oskar's hand, went with him to the bathroom.

'Don't cry,' I heard her say kindly as I hurried downstairs.

In the kitchen I half-filled a bucket with hot water, added some disinfectant, grabbed floor cloths and returned to Oskar's bedroom. As I cleaned the carpet, I could hear water running in the bathroom as the bath filled. Then Adrian's bedroom door opened. 'Is everything all right?' he asked.

'Yes, it's all under control,' I replied.

'Good.' And his door closed again.

But I was worried. Not because Oskar had had an accident, but because of the reason behind it. There was no doubt in my mind that seeing those toys had triggered a memory, which had caused him to wet himself. Children have accidents, but his expression had been one of pure terror. I'd had experience before of abused children having a flashback triggered by something apparently innocent, which had resulted in them losing control of their bladder and sometimes their bowels. I was convinced these toys meant far more than a reminder of home.

The water stopped running in the bathroom and Paula called, 'Mum, Oskar's bath is ready!'

'Thanks, love.' I left what I was doing and, taking Oskar's pyjamas from under his pillow, I went to the bathroom. Oskar was standing by the bath, still holding Paula's hand.

'Oskar, we'll wait outside while you take off your wet

clothes and pass them to me,' I said, giving him the privacy he needed. 'Then get into the bath.'

Paula and I waited on the landing with the door slightly ajar as Oskar undressed and then pushed his clothes through the gap. 'Thanks, love,' I said. 'Get into your bath and Paula will wait on the landing while I finish in your bedroom.'

Paula knew I waited on the landing every evening while Oskar had his bath. 'I won't be long,' I told her.

I put Oskar's clothes in the washing machine, then finished cleaning his bedroom carpet and patted it dry with clean cloths. I tipped away the dirty water and took the toys out of his room and put them in my bedroom. I thanked Paula for her help and took over.

As I waited for Oskar to finish his bath, I wondered how best to approach the subject of his toys, or if I should mention them at all. I would certainly make a note of Oskar's reaction in my log and advise Andrew, but what, if anything, should I say to Oskar? He was on the waiting list for therapy and the significance of the toys might come out then, but that could be months away.

I heard him get out of the bath, and once he'd dried himself and changed into his pyjamas he opened the bathroom door.

'Good boy. I'll fetch your dressing gown and you can come downstairs for a while. It's not your bedtime yet.'

'I'm tired,' he said. 'Can I go to bed now?'

'Yes, if you wish.' He looked tired and pale, I guessed from the upset.

I waited while he brushed his teeth and then went with him round the landing to his bedroom. 'I've put those toys away in my room for now,' I said. 'Was that the right thing to do?'

He nodded.

'Tell me if you want them.'

'I don't,' he said quietly. 'Not ever.'

He climbed into bed and snuggled down with his teddy bear, Luka, pulling the duvet right up to his chin. I looked at him. 'Oskar, love, is there anything you can tell me about those toys?'

He shook his head and screwed his eyes tightly shut, blocking me out.

'Tell me when you can, please. Goodnight, love.'

There was no reply, so I kissed his forehead and came out, drawing his door to behind me.

Downstairs I wrote up my log notes and then emailed Andrew:

> The bag of Oskar's belongings Mr Nowak left at school contained clothes and some new toys. Oskar seems fine about using the clothes but wants nothing to do with the toys. When he saw them he looked horrified and wet himself. I've put them away. Do you know who gave him those toys? Best wishes. Cathy

That night, Oskar had another nightmare and as usual I went straight to his room and sat with him until he was asleep again. I returned to my bed, where I lay awake worrying about him. How could I break through and release the demons that were taunting him? Just when I thought we were making progress, he closed down again. He needed to confide in someone, even if it wasn't me.

The following morning, tired from a broken night's sleep, I stumbled into our usual weekday routine. Oskar didn't mention the toys or the nightmare, but his expression said it all.

'Cheer up, Oskar, it might never happen,' Lucy said lightly as she passed him on the stairs.

Oskar looked even more downcast than normal this morning, while Lucy was in a permanent state of euphoria due, in part at least, I suspected, to her relationship with Darren. She'd never been a morning person, but now she was positively bouncy and couldn't wait to get to work. I just wished some of it could rub off on Oskar, but that wouldn't happen until he disclosed what was making him so sad. He ate his breakfast with the same gloomy expression and then I took him to school.

It was Tuesday, so we had contact that afternoon. Andrew hadn't replied to my email of the evening before, but it became obvious at the Family Centre that he had read it and acted upon it. Roksana was already in Green Room and it was clear from her expression she was angry with me.

'I don't know why you're making such a fuss,' she exclaimed as soon as we walked in. 'My friends give Oskar toys. What's wrong with that? When he has an accident he clears it up and puts his clothes in the washing machine. It's nothing to do with the toys. Why are you causing all this trouble?'

She made my worries sound almost farcical, as if I had completely overreacted. However, now wasn't the time for me to try to explain – in front of Oskar.

'I didn't intend to cause you any trouble,' I said. 'But it's probably best if we don't discuss it now.' I glanced at Oskar, who was looking anxiously at his mother.

Roksana huffed, clearly annoyed, but let the matter go. I hoped she wouldn't quiz Oskar about it during contact, and if she did that the contact supervisor would intervene and stop her. I said goodbye to them both and came away, now having doubts that I might have got it wrong. Perhaps the toys were innocent gifts and had nothing to do with Oskar wetting himself. A foster carer's life is full of doubts as we examine our actions, try to do our best and hope for good outcomes but realistically expect the worst.

When I collected Oskar, Roksana was cool with me but didn't say anything more about the toys. The evening continued as normal with dinner, Oskar reading, then a bath and bed. The following morning Oskar was quiet and pensive as usual. I took him to school, but then just before one o'clock, as I sat working at my computer, the house phone rang. It was the school secretary.

'Erica Jordan has asked me to call you,' she said. 'Can you come and collect Oskar, please? He's been crying all lunchtime but won't tell us what's wrong. She's with him now.'

'Yes, of course. I'll come straight away, although it will take me about fifteen minutes to get there.'

'That's fine. I'll let Miss Jordan know.'

Leaving the computer, I quickly pushed my feet into my shoes, grabbed my bag and went out the door. There are many reasons for a child being upset at school, including sickening for something, being bullied, fretting for their family, worrying about school, but usually a few kind words from a member of staff puts them right and I'm only told at the end of the day. Oskar was close to Miss Jordan and had confided in her before. That she hadn't been able to console him worried me even more.

A sickly feeling settled in my stomach as I parked the car outside the school and got out. It was lunchtime and the children were in the playground, running, laughing and playing – a complete contrast to what Oskar was going through. Because the children were in the playground the gate was security-locked, so I pressed the buzzer. It clicked open and I crossed the playground, weaving my way around the children. As I approached the main door it released. The school secretary would have seen me on the monitor in her office.

'Oskar is with his teacher in the medical room,' she said as I went in. 'It's down the corridor, third door on the left.'

I thanked her and headed along the corridor, my concerns growing. The school was strangely quiet with all the children playing outside. I knocked on the door of the medical room.

'Come in!' Miss Jordan called.

Oskar was sitting on a child's chair by the couch, while his teacher sat beside him on an adult chair. She had a box of tissues open on her lap. Although Oskar wasn't crying, he clearly had been; his eyes were red and his cheeks blotchy. He looked at me sadly.

'Thanks for coming,' Miss Jordan said. 'Oskar is feeling a bit better now he's been able to tell me what's wrong.'

'He's told you?' I asked. 'Thank goodness. What is it?' I went to him.

Oskar was staring down into his lap, twisting a tissue.

'He saw those two men in the black car parked outside at lunchtime. I'm so pleased he could tell me.'

'Yes, so am I. Well done, Oskar.' But he didn't appear greatly relieved from telling. 'The car isn't there now,' I added.

'No, I informed the Head straight away,' Miss Jordan said. 'She went out to speak to them, but they drove off when they saw her approaching. I believe she's telephoning Andrew.'

'Thank you.' I wondered if the reason they'd suddenly reappeared had anything to do with Roksana being upset and angry with me at contact for telling Andrew about Oskar's reaction to his toys.

'The Head said you could take Oskar home now rather than come back later if you wish.'

'I will, thank you. An afternoon off,' I said to Oskar with a smile. He didn't return it. Sombre and preoccupied, he slowly stood. 'You did well, telling Miss Jordan what upset you,' I said again, and Miss Jordan agreed.

She passed me Oskar's school bag and jacket and I thanked her for taking care of him. I said goodbye, that we'd see her tomorrow, and we left the medical room. In reception I told the school secretary I was taking Oskar home so she could amend their attendance record. We left the building and crossed the playground. The children were still playing during their lunch break, but Oskar was quiet and kept his head down.

'Are you OK, love?' I asked him, giving his hand a squeeze. He shrugged.

Oskar was quiet getting into the car and during the drive home, but when I parked outside the house he said, almost in a whisper, 'Cathy, you told me if there was anything worrying me, I should tell you.'

'Yes, that's right.' I turned in my seat so I could see him.

'I think I want to tell you something.' His face was pale and deadly serious.

'OK. Good. I'm listening.'

'Can we go in the house so no one can hear me?' he asked, looking anxiously through his side window.

There was no one around to hear, but he was obviously worried, so I got out, opened his car door and let us into the house. As soon as we were inside Oskar said, 'It's about those men in the car.'

'Yes. What about them?'

'I'm scared of them.'

'I know, love. Let's go and sit in the living room and you can tell me why. Do you want a drink of water?'

'No. I just want those men to leave me alone. They gave me toys and hurt me.'

I went ice cold and knew my worst fears were about to be realized.

CHAPTER FIFTEEN

THEY MADE ME

I now knew Oskar was going to tell me things I really didn't want to hear. Things that would keep me awake at night and haunt me for years to come, probably forever. Having heard previous foster children disclose abuse, I knew there were evil people in the world who were capable of anything and took advantage of innocent children for their own perverted pleasure. What's heard cannot be unheard. But if listening was bad, how much worse was it for the child who had suffered? I had to stay calm and strong for Oskar. It had taken a long time and a lot of courage for him to get to the point where he felt he could tell me, and he would need comfort and reassurance.

He and I sat on the sofa in the living room, side by side, Oskar's arm resting against mine. He reached out for my hand, so small and defenceless; a child's hand, in need of protection. Sammy was sitting at the patio window, gazing out down the garden, blissfully unaware of what was about to unfold. Oskar had fallen silent again, finding it difficult to begin.

'How did those men hurt you?' I asked after a moment.

'They did things to me.' His voice was slight, just above a whisper.

'What sort of things, love?'

'Rude things that hurt me.'

'Can you tell me what, so I can tell your social worker and the police?'

Another silence, then: 'Yes. They made me take off my pants. They touched my private parts and took photographs.' I felt physically sick and took a deep breath to steady myself.

'Both men did that?' I asked.

He nodded.

'The two men in the car?'

'Yes.'

'Were there ever any others present?'

'No.'

'Can you tell me the names of those two men?'

He shook his head.

'Can you write them down if I get a pen and paper?'

'No. They'll hurt me if I tell,' he said in the same tiny voice.

'Is that what they told you?'

'Yes.'

'They are very bad men, Oskar, but they can't hurt you any more.' I held his little hand between mine. 'You're safe now.'

'I don't think I am,' he said, his voice quivering. 'They said they'd find me if I told and cut me up in little bits, but I had to tell you because I'm unhappy all the time.'

'I know, love.' I put my arm around him. 'You've done the right thing. They won't harm you again,' I said firmly, blinking back my tears. 'They won't be coming anywhere near you, ever. Did you tell your mother what they did?'

He shook his head. 'They said if I told her or anyone, they'd cut her up in little bits too. But I've told you. Will they come and get you, me and Mummy?' He looked at me, petrified.

'No, they won't. Absolutely not. I can promise you that. They won't hurt you or any of us. They will be going to prison for a long time.'

'I'm scared,' he said, shivering. 'They gave me toys and said I mustn't tell, but I don't want the toys.'

'I know. I've put them away. You've done the right thing to tell me.'

'When I saw the toys, it made me remember how they hurt me,' he said. 'That's why I wet myself.'

'I understand. They are very bad men and they will be punished. You won't be hurt again.'

His hand trembled in mine as he struggled to say more. 'Sometimes I wet myself when they were doing bad things to me and they laughed.'

I swallowed hard. 'They are evil,' I said, trying to hold back my anger.

'I had to bend over so they could take photos of my bottom and willy. I knew it was wrong, but I couldn't stop them.' He began to cry.

I held him close. I went to speak but my voice caught in my throat. It was a moment before I could ask, 'Where did all this happen?'

'In my house when I got home from school. I used to hate going home from school. I wanted to stay with Miss Jordan.'

'Was Uncle Nowak there?' I knew he'd often collected Oskar from school.

'No. He took me home and then left for work. Whoever was in the house was supposed to look after me. But there wasn't anyone in after school but those men. Everyone else was working. It was just me and them until dinnertime.'

'How often did they do this to you?' I asked. It was important I gathered as much information as possible while

Oskar was talking so I could tell Andrew and ultimately the police.

'Lots of times,' he said, shuddering. 'It got worse when Mummy was away and went to see Luka. They hit me, that's how I got the bruise on my face.'

'And your mother didn't know?' I asked again.

'No.'

'You've done well to tell me, Oskar. Is there anything else you want to tell me now?'

'I didn't want to do it,' he said, stifling another sob. 'They made me. They said it was a game and I liked to play it. But I didn't, honestly. It wasn't my fault, was it?' He looked up at me beseechingly and I could have wept.

'No. It certainly wasn't your fault,' I said firmly. 'None of it was. Bad men like that tell the child they are abusing it's a game and they enjoy it. They give them gifts and threaten them, which makes the child very confused, so it's more difficult for them to tell. You've been very brave, Oskar. I am proud of you.'

'Will my mummy be proud of me?' he asked quietly.

'She certainly should be,' I replied. But I knew from experience that parents reacted differently to being told their child had been abused while in their care. Some believed the child unreservedly, supported them and ostracized the abuser, even separating from a partner if it was them. Others refused to believe the child had been abused and claimed they were lying, which was devastating for the child and often impacted on them for the rest of their life.

Oskar and I were silent, the enormity of what he'd disclosed thick in the air. I then realized I had my arm around him and he'd been letting me hold and comfort him, something he'd never allowed me to do before. I stayed where I was, still and quiet, the weight of his little body against mine. I needed to phone Andrew, but that could wait for a few more minutes.

'I like hugs,' I said softly after a moment.

'So do I,' he said and, slipping his arm around my waist, he hugged me for all he was worth. It was our first proper hug and it had taken the disclosure of dreadful abuse to allow him to do it.

'Mummy doesn't have time for hugs,' he said presently, and a tear escaped and ran down my cheek. After all the hurt he'd described, it was something as simple as this that had finally made me cry. I wiped away the tear and swallowed hard.

'Hopefully she will in the future,' I said unevenly, and held him closer still.

I knew that all the signs Oskar had been sexually abused had been there from the beginning: not wanting to take off his clothes, the nightmares, his wariness around men, being permanently anxious and sad. And all those times when he'd started to tell me something and, out of fear of being cut up, had stopped. Oskar had said the toys from home had hurt him, but I could now see what he meant. It wasn't the toys themselves; it was that he associated being hurt with the toys.

I also remembered how cautious he'd been when I'd first given him the teddy bear I'd bought. Now I understood that presents in the past had been given to buy his silence. Whatever had gone through his mind when I'd given him what I thought was an innocent present? Little wonder he'd been wary of us, especially Adrian. Before I telephoned Andrew and he set the wheels in motion, I needed to try to begin to restore Oskar's faith in others, although I was sure it would take years before he truly trusted anyone again. One of the lasting legacies of sexual abuse is distrust.

'Oskar, those two men who abused you were evil – very, very bad, wicked men – but most men aren't evil. They're good. Adrian is a good person. He won't hurt you, and neither will your social worker. You have nothing to fear from them or most men.' Obvious to those from loving homes who haven't suffered, but not to an abused child. 'I'm going to telephone your social worker now and tell him what you've told me. OK, love?'

Oskar reluctantly took his arms from around me. 'We can have another hug when I've finished,' I said with a smile. 'Would you like to watch some television while I talk to Andrew?'

'Yes, please,' he said quietly.

'Good boy.'

I switched on the television, found a children's channel, then, taking my mobile, I stepped outside the living room, drawing the door slightly to. With the television on, Oskar shouldn't be able to hear me. I tapped Andrew's office number and he answered straight away.

'Sorry, I was going to phone you,' he said. 'Elaine Summer called and said Oskar was upset. I understand he saw those two men again parked outside his school.'

'Yes, that's right. I've brought Oskar home, but there's been a development since then.' I told Andrew everything Oskar had told me, finishing with, 'I've no doubt Oskar is telling me the truth.'

There was a moment's pause and then Andrew said, with a heartfelt sigh, 'I agree. The poor child. I'll alert the police straight away. How is he?'

'Very quiet. He's watching some television. I've reassured him as much as I can.'

'I'll need to see him at some point, but let me get this moving first. Did he say if anyone else knew of the abuse?'

'From what he said it was just him and those two men in the house at the time of the abuse. I don't think anyone else knew.'

'And he wouldn't give you their names?'

'No, he's too scared.'

'And he didn't tell his mother?'

'He says not.'

'Do we know when the abuse started?'

'I didn't ask him, but I got the feeling it was weeks if not months ago. It escalated when Roksana was out of the country, seeing Luka.'

'Because there was no one in the house responsible for Oskar,' Andrew said. 'Roksana told me her friends were looking after him while she worked and was away, but clearly that wasn't so. OK, thank you, Cathy. I'll be in touch.'

'Andrew, one more thing. There is supposed to be phone contact this evening. Do you want Oskar to call his mother?'

He paused for a moment and then said, 'No. I don't want her alerted until the police have been to the house and spoken to her.'

'All right.'

The call ended and I returned to the living room. Oskar was where I'd left him, sitting on the sofa facing the television, although I'm not sure he was actually watching the programme. As soon as I entered, he turned and looked at me, worried. 'Did you tell Andrew?' he asked anxiously.

'Yes. He will tell the police. You've been very brave. There is nothing for you to worry about now.'

'I hope the police catch those men and lock them up,' he said in the innocent, childish way of a six-year-old.

'So do I,' I said. 'It would help if you could tell me their names.'

But I could see from his expression he was still too scared to tell, and he slowly shook his head.

'OK. I'm sure the police will be able to find out who they are,' I said with a reassuring smile. 'You're safe. Nothing can harm you now.' I'd said it before and I would say it again, many times, although I knew it would be a long time before he truly felt safe.

I left Oskar briefly again while I fetched my fostering folder from the locked draw in the front room. I wanted to write up my log notes while what Oskar had told me was still fresh in my mind. It was possible my log would form part of the evidence against the two men when they were caught. So while Oskar continued to watch the television, I sat a little way from him on the sofa and wrote what had happened that day – from when the school secretary had telephoned to what Oskar had told his teacher and his disclosure to me, using his words as much as possible. I ended by writing that I had telephoned his social worker at 3 p.m. and notified him.

I returned the folder to the drawer in the front room and sat beside Oskar again. Now all I could do was wait and hope that those two men were caught and there was enough evidence to prosecute them. Sadly, I'd fostered children before who had found the courage to disclose abuse, but then after a police investigation there'd been insufficient evidence to take the case to court. Not only was it frustrating for all those involved with the child, but it was soul-destroying for the child or young person who hadn't seen their abuser punished. Having said that, I know some victims have found that being able to tell and having their claims taken seriously and investigated by the police has given them some closure.

I looked at Oskar as he watched television, his little face so innocent and vulnerable. It beggared belief how anyone could hurt and humiliate him. My anger flared towards those responsible and I felt even more protective of him. I wondered how Roksana would feel when she was told what had happened. There was nothing so far to suggest she knew Oskar was being abused, but she'd repeatedly left him without proper supervision, so that when she'd worked and gone abroad he'd been at the mercy of two paedophiles. However, there was no point in speculating, for now my priority was – as always – Oskar.

'How are you doing?' I asked him after a moment, touching his arm.

He gave a little nod and turned to look at me. 'I feel a bit better now I've told you,' he said, and managed a small smile. I could have cried.

'Good. I thought you might.'

'Can I have another hug?' he asked.

'Yes, of course.' I put my arm around him and he snuggled close. We continued watching television, hugging each other. It was at moments like this I knew exactly why I fostered. I had helped Oskar take the first step towards a better future.

As Paula, Lucy and Adrian returned home I took them aside and told them that Oskar had disclosed sexual abuse (although not the details) and if he said anything else they should let me know so I could pass it on to his social worker. Sometimes when a child starts to talk about the abuse they've suffered more comes tumbling out, and it was important I logged it and told the social worker, as it was all evidence. Of course, my children were horrified that Oskar had been abused, although they weren't wholly surprised. Having grown up with fostering, they could often spot the signs when a child was harbouring a dark secret, just as I could. Fostering had taught us that evil things do happen and they're not just horror stories in the news.

It was only as we sat down to dinner that Oskar realized he hadn't telephoned his mother.

'Andrew decided we wouldn't call her today, as he'll need to talk to her and she'll have a lot on her mind,' I said.

'Oh, I like talking to her,' he said, disappointed. Which surprised me, as they struggled to make conversation and the calls were never more than a couple of minutes. I supposed it was the brief contact with his mother and hearing her voice that he liked. I didn't doubt he loved her, and she him, but Roksana's absence during so much of his life due to her long working hours had prevented them from forming a very close attachment.

That night, unsurprisingly, Oskar had another nightmare. When I went to his room I found him trying to fight someone off and shouting, 'Don't hurt me!' It didn't take much to guess who. I reassured him he was safe and, once he was in a deep sleep again, I returned to my bedroom. I was sure Oskar would have more nightmares while his subconscious purged itself of the dreadful memories of abuse, until he could finally sleep peacefully.

CHAPTER SIXTEEN

QUESTIONED BY THE POLICE

Oskar didn't want to go to school the following morning, which hadn't happened before, as he liked school. After sitting with him in his bedroom for some time and encouraging him to tell me why, he confessed he was worried that, now he'd told, those two men would come to his school and cut him into little pieces. I told him that was impossible, that the building was security-locked and protected by CCTV; his teacher would make sure he was safe and those men would probably be in police custody by now, so they couldn't harm him.

'If I go to school, I don't want to go in the playground,' he said. 'They might get over the fence.'

The fencing was over six feet high, but I said, 'Would it help if I spoke to Miss Jordan and see what she suggests?'

'Yes,' he said in a tiny voice. He had faith in her.

Now partially reassured, Oskar got dressed, had some breakfast, then sat quietly, deep in thought, in the back of the car as I drove to his school. As we walked along the pavement towards the building I could see him looking round, scanning the parked cars for any sign of the black car, as indeed I was, although I didn't tell him that. Instead, I pointed out the high fencing, security-locked main gate, the CCTV and the playground supervisor, trying to reassure him. However, as he was worried, I didn't wait in the playground for the start of school but went straight to the main door and pressed the bell. The secretary let us in.

Elaine Summer, the Head, was in reception and greeted us with a warm smile and bright, 'Good morning. How are you today?' – mainly directed at Oskar, so I wondered if she was aware of what had happened after I'd taken him home yesterday lunchtime. Oskar was subdued and looking at me to say something about his concerns.

'Oskar is worried that those two men in the car might come into the school to get him.'

'Certainly not. I telephoned your social worker yesterday as soon as you told your teacher they were outside. He's dealing with it,' Elaine replied.

'Things have moved on since then,' I said. 'Have you spoken to Andrew since then?'

'No.' She frowned, puzzled.

We were alone in reception and, as the Head Teacher, she needed to know. 'When I took Oskar home yesterday, he was brave enough to tell me that the two men in the car had abused him while he'd been living with them and his mother.' Elaine's face fell and she instinctively touched Oskar's shoulder in a gesture of protectiveness.

'Have they been arrested?' she asked me quietly.

'I don't know yet. I'm waiting to hear from Andrew.'

'We'll keep a look-out,' Elaine said to Oskar, and she smiled at him. Then to me: 'Even if they're not in custody yet, they're unlikely to return here if the police are looking for them.'

I agreed, but Oskar said, 'Please, Miss, I don't want to go in the playground.'

'No. All right. You can stay inside for today. We'll look after you.'

'Thank you,' I said. Oskar looked relieved too.

'Would you like to come and sit in my office until school starts?' she asked Oskar. This was clearly a privilege and he nodded enthusiastically.

I thanked the Head again and left Oskar in her capable hands. As I walked away it occurred to me that she had previously seen the two men close up when she'd spoken to them when they'd been waiting outside the school. I assumed, if it was necessary, she could probably give a good description of them to the police.

I was expecting to hear from Andrew, but at 12.15 Miss Jordan telephoned. My first thought was that something bad had happened or that Oskar was very upset and needed to be collected. But thankfully she said, 'I wanted to let you know Oskar is doing all right.' I breathed a sigh of relief. 'He stayed indoors with me during morning play and is now having some lunch. He's going outside with the other children once he's finished eating, but the playground supervisor has been informed and will be looking out for him.'

'Thank you so much,' I said.

'You're welcome. I thought you'd be worrying about him. I know I do.'

She was a treasure.

'Have they caught those men yet?' Miss Jordan asked. 'The Head told me what Oskar said about them. I was so upset and angry.'

'I haven't heard any more. I'm hoping his social worker will phone before too long.'

'Oh dear. Well, don't worry, we're looking after Oskar.'

I thanked her again and said I'd be in the playground at the end of school as usual to collect him.

Oskar was due to see his mother that afternoon and I needed to know if contact was going ahead, so when I still hadn't heard from Andrew at two o'clock I called his office. A colleague answered and I gave my name and said I was Oskar's foster carer. She told me Andrew was out of the office and she didn't know when he'd be back. I emphasized that I needed to know if contact was going ahead today, and she said she'd telephone Andrew and ask him to call me. 'I'll need to know within the hour,' I added. 'I collect Oskar from school and take him straight to the Family Centre.'

Over an hour later, as I parked outside Oskar's school, my mobile rang and it was Andrew. 'I got your message,' he said, clearly in a hurry. 'Yes, contact will go ahead as normal today.'

'Thank you. And phone contact tomorrow?'

'Yes.'

It didn't seem as though he was going to say any more, so I asked, 'Have those two men been identified?'

'They have. Roksana and others living at the same address were able to give their names to the police.'

'Good. Have they been arrested? Oskar is very concerned they might come after him at school.'

'No. They didn't return to the house last night. It seems someone might have alerted them.' Which wasn't good news. 'The police are looking for them. I'll need to see Oskar as soon as I can. I'll be in touch.'

'OK. Thank you.' And the call ended.

I wouldn't tell Oskar the men hadn't been caught; indeed, I wouldn't mention it at all unless he did. As I walked towards the school I automatically looked up and down the road for any sign of the black car, although realistically they weren't going to risk returning here now they knew they were wanted by the police. But it didn't stop me glancing over my shoulder as I waited in the playground.

When Oskar's class came out he was with Miss Jordan and she came over with him. His face had lost some of its anxiety, so I guessed he'd had a good day and was perhaps enjoying the extra attention. 'He's been fine all day,' Miss Jordan said. 'I'm very proud of him.' Oskar smiled. 'Is there any news?' she asked me.

I shook my head. I could see Oskar watching me. 'We're going to contact now.'

'Really?' she asked, surprised, perhaps thinking that contact would have been stopped.

'Contact is going ahead as usual,' I confirmed. 'We'll see you tomorrow. Thank you so much for looking after Oskar.'

'I hope it goes well,' she said, not wholly reassured that seeing his mother was in Oskar's best interests.

I had reservations too. But it takes a lot to stop contact, as it's part of the court order set by the judge.

'I hope my mummy isn't angry with me,' Oskar said as we walked to the car.

'For what?'

'Telling on those men.'

'You did the right thing,' I said, and quietly hoped Roksana thought so too.

'Roksana is here,' the receptionist said as Oskar and I entered the Family Centre. 'She was early. You're in Red Room today. The contact supervisor has just gone in.'

I thank her, signed the Visitors' Book, and Oskar held my hand as we went along the corridor.

'Why's the room changed?' he asked.

'I'm not sure, it does sometimes, but all the rooms are nice.'

The door to Red Room was slightly open, but I knocked anyway before we went in. The same contact supervisor was seated at the table with a notebook and pen ready. Roksana was sitting on the sofa, not checking her phone as she usually was, but staring into space. She looked dreadful, pale and drawn. As soon as she saw us, she stood and, with a small cry, rushed over. 'Are you all right?' she asked Oskar, enfolding him in her arms.

I could see he was as surprised as I was by her unusual display of affection. I don't think I'd ever seen her hug him or even touch him before.

He stood awkwardly, arms by his side and rigid, unable to respond to his mother. There were tears in Roksana's eyes. 'Are you all right?' I asked her, gently going over.

'Not really,' she said, and, releasing Oskar, she began to cry openly. Oskar had had his question answered: his mother wasn't angry, but very upset.

He went to the table and brought back the box of tissues and gave one to her.

'Thank you,' she said between sobs.

'Don't cry, Mummy,' he said in a small voice, looking at her anxiously.

'I'm sorry,' she said, trying to stem her tears.

'Would you like a few minutes by yourself?' I asked her. 'We could wait outside.'

'No. I want him near me. I've phoned in sick at work. I couldn't face it, but I told Andrew I'd be all right at contact.'

She wiped her eyes, blew her nose and gradually composed herself. 'Sorry,' she said again.

'It's OK.'

'I'm all right,' she told Oskar and the contact supervisor. I guessed he'd never seen his mother upset before; she always appeared strong. Then to me she said, 'I know I'm not allowed to talk to Oskar about what he said, but can I phone you later, please?'

'Yes, I don't see why not.' Carers are expected to work with the child's parents as much as possible. I'd note her call in my log and pass on to Andrew anything he needed to know. However, Roksana hadn't to be given my contact details.

'I could phone you later,' I suggested.

'Yes, please.'

'Around eight o'clock if that suits you,' I said, so that it would be after Oskar was in bed.

'Yes. I'm not working this evening.'

Oskar was still looking worried. 'Come on, love, your mother is going to be OK now. Let's find a game for you two to play.'

As Roksana finished wiping her eyes, I took Oskar to the shelves containing the boxes of puzzles and games. He chose a couple of puzzles and carried them to the sofa. Roksana joined him, and I left them sitting together, with Oskar slowly removing a game from its box. He wasn't showing much enthusiasm and I knew contact was going to be difficult for both of them, but at least they were together for an hour.

When I returned to collect Oskar, he and his mother were still sitting side by side on the sofa, and unlike at previous contacts she didn't appear in any hurry to leave, presumably because she wasn't going to work. They were talking quietly, it seemed about Oskar's school, and I wondered how often in the past they'd just sat and talked. I doubted it was much, for Roksana was always rushing from one job to another, leaving Oskar in the care of whoever had been in the house. I waited inside the door and it was a few moments before Roksana said to Oskar, 'I think you have to go now, unless Cathy can come back later.'

I saw the contact supervisor glance over, though she left it to me to explain. 'I'm afraid we have to keep to the time set,' I said. 'But you could ask Andrew if contact could be extended in the future.' Andrew had originally offered Roksana longer, but she'd refused because of her work commitments.

'I'll have to see if I can change my shift,' she said.

I nodded.

'You go with Cathy then,' she told Oskar, 'and I'll see what I can do.'

He immediately stood and came to me. 'Would you like to give your mother a kiss goodbye?' I suggested. Usually it's not necessary for me to say this, as children naturally want to kiss and cuddle their parents at the end of contact, but Roksana and Oskar had never done that. They weren't tactile. Oskar dutifully returned to his mother and kissed her cheek. She immediately welled up but didn't kiss him back.

'I'm sorry I've not been a better mother,' she said, taking a tissue from the box.

Oskar clearly didn't know what to say, so he gave his mother another kiss and came to me. 'I'll phone you at eight,' I told Roksana.

'Yes, please.' She nodded and blew her nose. 'Here's my new number. The police have my old phone.' I accepted the piece of paper she passed to me, and Oskar and I left.

Oskar was having to deal with his own emotions and really needed to see his mother strong, although I understood why she couldn't be at present. Finding out that Oskar had been abused by people she trusted had clearly come as a huge shock. But in the vast majority of these cases, children are abused by someone they know. Stranger danger is rare. It's usually someone the parents know and trust – a relative, friend or neighbour. Paedophiles are devious in gaining the trust of a parent and often target single parents, taking time to build a relationship with them and their family before they strike.

I waited until Oskar was in bed and asleep before I telephoned Roksana. I sat in the living room with the door closed. Paula was in her bedroom and Adrian and Lucy were out, although they wouldn't be late back, as they had work in the morning. It was exactly eight o'clock as I pressed Roksana's number. She answered straight away. 'It's Cathy.'

'Oh, thank you so much for calling. I don't know what to do,' she said and burst into tears. 'I'm sorry, I'm in a dreadful state,' she continued through stifled sobs. 'My solicitor can't see me until next week. I don't think I'll ever get Oskar back now and my sister says it's my fault. I don't see any point in –'

'Roksana,' I interrupted. 'I know this has come as a dreadful shock, but don't lose hope. No one is accusing you of abusing Oskar or knowing he was being abused. He told me more than once that he didn't tell you and I passed that on to Andrew.'

'Thank you. But I feel I am to blame. I should have been more careful who I left him with. I know that's what the police thought – that I was a bad mother for leaving him, but I had to.'

'Were you interviewed by the police?' I asked.

'Yes, everyone in the house was. They raided us at five o'clock this morning. Some of us were still in bed. They questioned us all, but Mihai and Codrin had gone. I don't know where they are now.'

'Mihai and Codrin are the two men who abused Oskar?' I asked.

'Yes. I told the police their names, but I don't know any more about them. Mihai was a friend of someone who lived in the house last year. When he and Codrin turned up needing somewhere to live we had a spare room, so we let them have it. That often happens here. People come and go, and we have to fill the house to pay the bills and send money home. They seemed OK, but I didn't know them before they came to live with us. How was I to know they were perverts?' She paused, again overcome with emotion.

Obviously, Roksana couldn't have known they were 'perverts' – paedophiles are often outwardly as normal as the average person – but her mistake was to leave Oskar with people she didn't know, which she now realized.

'I've never been in trouble with the police before,' she continued through her tears. 'We are all under suspicion and they have taken our iPads and smartphones. I feel like a criminal. I've had to buy a cheap phone, as I need it for work and calling my sister and Luka.'

'It's normal procedure to take these devices,' I said. 'The police will return them to you once they've finished with them.'

'Yes, that's what they said. I feel dirty. How am I ever going to get Oskar back now? I honestly had no idea he was being abused or I would have done something. Why didn't he tell me?'

'He was too scared. They threatened him and it took him a long time to tell me,' I said diplomatically. But, of course, Roksana needed to have been there, with time to listen, ask the right questions and coax it out of him, which she hadn't been. Not that I was blaming her, but Oskar might have been

able to confide in his mother if they'd had a closer relationship. Since publishing my fostering memoirs, sadly I've heard
from many adults who were abused as children and tried to
tell, but either weren't listened to or weren't believed.

'How is Oskar?' Roksana finally thought to ask. 'He
seemed OK at contact.'

'I doubt he's OK,' I said. 'I think there's a lot going on
inside that he's keeping a tight lid on at present.'

'You don't think there's more?' she asked, horrified.

'I don't know, but even if there's not, it will take time for
Oskar to heal emotionally. It will be nice if you can spend
more time with him at contact. Did you ask Andrew?'

'No, it's not possible,' she said. 'I phoned the agency and I
can't change my evening shift. Oskar won't mind.'

These words made me wonder just how much Roksana
had learnt from what had happened and how far she was
willing to change to try to win back custody of her son.

CHAPTER SEVENTEEN

SICKENING

Roksana had been right when she'd said Oskar appeared to be OK. He did outwardly, but I knew the hurt and anger from the abuse would be bubbling inside him. No one who has been abused walks away unscathed. His turmoil would surface eventually, one way or another.

The next day and during that weekend Oskar was his usual quiet and contained little self, although he did want plenty of hugs from me, and then Lucy and Paula. We were of course happy to oblige. He was still wary around Adrian and I hoped that in time this would pass as his trust in men was restored. Therapy should help, but I was still waiting for an appointment for CAMHS.

When we telephoned Roksana in the evening the conversation between her and Oskar was as short and stilted as before. I don't think she knew how to talk to her son – she never really had. I prompted Oskar to tell his mother about school and what he'd been doing generally, but she replied to everything with a flat, 'That's nice.' It sounded dismissive and didn't invite further conversation, although I don't think she meant it to. It was her way with Oskar. I also thought she must have a lot on her mind, dealing with Oskar's disclosure and the police investigation. But at least she held it together while she spoke to him on the phone and didn't cry. Had she, I would have stopped the phone call, as it would have been upsetting for Oskar.

On Monday Andrew telephoned mid-morning and said that the police were going to video interview Oskar that afternoon and he would collect him from school at one-thirty, take him to the interview and then return him to me afterwards. I was relieved Andrew was taking Oskar rather than me. I'd accompanied other children I'd fostered to similar interviews and knew how upsetting it could be. The police are specially trained to interview young children and are sensitive to their needs, but obviously they have to ask in-depth questions to obtain enough detail to prosecute the abuser(s). The interview is usually conducted in a special suite at the police station with a sofa and toys, designed to relax the child. For the actual interview, just the child and interviewing officer are present, but there is an adjacent room where the person accompanying the child can wait and observe what happens. Watching and listening to a child describe the details of sexual abuse stays with you for years to come, although I'd already heard some of what Oskar had suffered when he'd disclosed to me. I think foster carers should be offered counselling. Some fostering agencies do but not all, and it relies on the carer's supervising social worker to apply for it, when it should come as standard.

That afternoon my thoughts were with Oskar. As one-thirty approached I began worrying about him and continued to do so all afternoon. It was nearly five o'clock before Andrew returned him and they both looked washed out. 'I'll come in briefly,' Andrew said. 'Then I need to stop by the office.'

'Are you OK?' I asked Oskar.

He nodded. 'I'm going to my room,' he said, and kicking off his shoes he went upstairs. Paula was in her room so I asked her to keep an eye on him while I talked to Andrew.

Andrew gratefully accepted a coffee, which I set on a tray with a plate of biscuits and carried into the living room. I placed it on the occasional table within his reach. 'Thank you,' he said, and with a heartfelt sigh he took a few sips. 'Oskar did well. The police should have enough evidence with his testimony and the evidence they found in the house to prosecute those responsible, once they catch them.'

'They haven't caught Mihai and Codrin yet?'

'No, and it's unlikely those were their real names, but the police know who they are from the details given by those in the house. They've told Oskar they are looking for them and have reassured him he is safe and they won't come after him.'

'Good. He was worried they might.'

'I know, he told the police he was.' Andrew took another sip from his coffee. 'I'm going to speak to CAMHS and try to bring forward Oskar's appointment. I think it should be classified as urgent now.'

'Yes. That would help him. I'm glad there's enough evidence to prosecute.'

'So am I,' Andrew said, setting down his cup. 'The police found a number of USB memory sticks concealed in a mattress in the room they used. They'd recorded some of the abuse as it took place.'

My stomach churned. I didn't ask what was on those USB sticks, I could guess. Unbelievably sick and shocking clips of children being abused, destined to be shared with other paedophiles on the Dark Web. This is a place on the Internet most of us are completely unaware of, as it won't come up on a search engine, but it's where criminals – paedophiles, terrorists, traffickers and so forth – share their illegal activities.

'The recordings showed other children being abused as well as Oskar,' Andrew said. 'The police are trying to identify and trace them. There is nothing to suggest that Roksana or anyone else living in the house knew or was involved, although the police enquiries are on-going.'

I nodded. Obviously, it was a relief that his mother wasn't involved.

'I'd better be going,' Andrew said with a sigh, and finished his coffee. 'Can you let me have a copy of your log notes? Anything that relates to Oskar disclosing abuse.'

'Yes, of course. I'll type them up this evening. Is Oskar to phone his mother tonight?'

'Yes, contact is as usual. I'll go up and say goodbye to him and leave you to it.'

I waited in the hall while Andrew went up to Oskar's room and Paula left them together. After he'd gone, I went to check on Oskar. He was sitting on his bed. 'Are you all right?'

'Yes,' he said in a small voice.

'Andrew tells me you did very well.'

'I didn't tell the police their names,' he said seriously. 'Someone else did.'

'I know. There's nothing for you to worry about.'

'Will they know it wasn't me?' he asked anxiously.

'I don't know, but it doesn't matter. Those evil men won't come anywhere near you. They are wanted by the police and on the run. They will be far away from here by now.' I hoped I was right. The last thing Oskar needed was to see them again, even from a distance. 'You have to phone your mother, so let's go downstairs now and do that.'

'Will she want to speak to me?' he asked gloomily.

'Yes, of course. Although it's later than we usually phone so she may be at work. If she doesn't answer you can leave a message.' That he had to ask was worrying, as most children would assume their parent wanted to talk to them.

Downstairs in the living room, we sat in our usual places side by side on the sofa and, with the phone on speaker, I pressed Roksana's number. As I thought might happen, the call went through to voicemail. 'Leave Mummy a message,' I told Oskar, and passed him the phone.

'Hello, Mummy,' he said in a small voice. 'It's Oskar.' And that was it. He handed the phone back to me.

'It's Cathy,' I said. 'Hope you're OK. I'm guessing you're at work, so we'll see you tomorrow at contact. Just to let you know that Oskar is all right. Bye, then.'

I kept Oskar occupied that evening. He fed Sammy and then helped me make dinner. He didn't want much to eat and kept yawning at the table, so I guessed he was exhausted from the afternoon. I took him up for an early bath and bed. As I tucked him into bed he asked, 'Will those men be a long way away now?'

'Yes. Don't worry.'

'How do you know?'

'Andrew told me the police were looking for them. I think they told you something similar?'

'Yes, but how do they know they have gone?' he persisted.

'The police are smart,' I said. 'They know all about catching criminals.'

'Smarter than those men?' he asked.

'Yes, much smarter.' Which seemed to help. At Oskar's age, he was simply looking for reassurance, and didn't need to know the ins and outs of a police enquiry.

I sat with him for a while and then, kissing his forehead, I left him to go to sleep, which he did quite quickly. Downstairs I took my log book and a marker pen from the drawer in the front room and sat at the table, going through my notes, highlighting all the sections relevant to Oskar disclosing abuse. Not just the actual time he'd managed to tell me but when he'd got close, and how he'd been – if he'd gone quiet and appeared anxious. It would help build a case and substantiate what he was saying. Once I'd finished going through my log book, I typed the extracts into a Word document and emailed it to Andrew.

Afterwards I spent time with my children, all of whom were in, and then went to bed, finally falling asleep in the early hours. Oskar slept well and seemed refreshed in the morning. However, as we left the house to go to school I got the shock of my life. He was just ahead of me on the front path and as he approached our gate he suddenly screamed and darted round the corner of the house, terrified. I went after him, my heart racing, and found him crouching behind a large potted shrub down the sideway.

'Whatever is the matter?' I asked. 'Have you been stung?' It was my first thought as the rhododendron bush in the front garden was in flower and wasps were buzzing around it.

'They're there!' he cried, burying his head in his knees and pointing to the road. 'I saw their car.'

I felt sick with fear. I didn't need him to tell me who. 'Stay there,' I said, and quickly took out my phone ready to call the police. I returned to our garden gate and saw what was frightening Oskar. A black car was parked on the opposite side of the road, but it was a different make and model to the one his abusers had, and this car was empty. True, it wasn't usually parked there, but there were any number of reasons why it could be, and there was nothing to link it to his abusers other than its colour.

'It's not them,' I said, putting away my phone as I returned to him. 'It's a different car. It belongs to someone else.'

'Are you sure?' he asked, daring to raise his head.

'Yes, positive.' I offered him my hand and he slowly came out from his hiding place. 'See,' I said as we went to the gate and the car came into view. 'It's very different and it's empty.'

'But why is it here?' he asked.

'The owner is probably visiting someone who lives in the road. It's nothing to worry about.'

I opened his car door and he got in, but I could see he was still looking anxiously across the road. 'Oskar, there are thousands of black cars. It's one of the most popular colours. I'll show you on the way to school.'

I started the car and pulled away, then as I drove I pointed out all the black cars I could see, and there were plenty! 'There's one,' I said. 'There's another one ...' And so on, until I felt I had made my point. 'OK?' I asked, glancing at him in the rear-view mirror.

'Yes.' But a few moments later he said, 'Their car smelt funny inside.'

My heart stopped and I had a sinking feeling in the pit of my stomach. There was only one way he could know that. 'Have you been in their car?' I asked.

'Yes.'

'Were you abused in their car?'

I saw him nod.

'Did you tell the police?' I kept my eyes on the road ahead.

'Yes. I told them everything.'

'Good boy.'

Oskar was quiet for the rest of the journey to school while I struggled with the images and thoughts racing through my head. Not only of Oskar being abused at home and in their car, but of the other children the police had discovered on those sickening videos. It was horrendous, and I only knew part of what had happened. It was enough to strike terror into the hearts of any caring adult. I wondered if the parents of the other children in the videos knew they had been abused or possibly still were being. It's the stuff of nightmares, and hearing about it undermines one's faith in human nature. There are evil people out there. Oskar was safe, but what about all the others? It's a shocking thought that thousands of children across the world are being abused at this very moment.

On a lighter note, when we arrived in the school playground, fellow foster carer Angela came over. I hadn't seen her for a while and I soon learnt why. She'd been involved in rehabilitating the brother and sister she was fostering back home to their mother, so for the last few weeks the children had been attending their new school, near their home. Angela had brought them here today to say goodbye to their class. While it was fantastic the children could go home, it was bittersweet for Angela, who, like most foster carers, had grown very close to them. We talked for a while and then, when it was time for the children to go into school, we said goodbye. It was unlikely we'd see each other at the end of the day as Oskar and I had to leave smartly to go to contact and she would be involved in final goodbyes. I'd probably see her again at a foster-carer training or one of the social events.

Later, as I drove to contact that afternoon, I wondered if I'd ever be in the same position as Angela and returning Oskar home. I thought it unlikely. A lot would have to change before the social services felt it safe to return him. Roksana hadn't abused her son, but her neglect had left him without proper parenting and vulnerable to abuse.

As if to give weight to my supposition, Roksana was late for contact. She'd phoned the Family Centre to say she was on her way, so Oskar and I waited in Green Room with the contact supervisor for her to arrive. I read story books to Oskar to pass the time.

'Sorry,' she said, when she finally appeared twenty minutes late. 'I didn't sleep well and my boss is angry I phoned in sick yesterday. Bastard. It's the first time I've ever been off sick.' She looked tired and strained.

'That doesn't seem fair,' I said sympathetically. 'Can't you work for a different agency?' I knew there were plenty of cleaning agencies in the area.

'I'll have to if he fires me,' she said, dumping her bag and jacket on the sofa. 'But they pay better than most agencies.'

I returned the books we'd been reading to the shelf. 'Have a good time with Oskar.'

'Oh yes, Oskar,' she said, as if seeing him for the first time. She'd been so preoccupied with her work worries that he'd come second again. I wondered again if she'd truly learnt any lessons from what had happened.

Outside, I sat in my car with the window down and the radio on. It wasn't worth going home. Presently my phone bleeped with a text message from Lucy: *Hi Mum. I'm going to spend the night at Darren's. See you tomorrow.* 😃

Oh no you're not! was my first thought. Then I stopped and took a moment.

This had caught me unawares. I hadn't realized their relationship had progressed so quickly and, in my eyes, Lucy was still my little girl, just as Paula was. I took a breath and tried to think rationally. Adrian spent nights with Kirsty, but they'd known each other for years, not weeks, and, dare I say it, Adrian was more sensible – his head ruled his heart. Lucy was the opposite, but I loved her for it. I'd seen the way her face lit up every time she mentioned Darren, which was often. She was besotted with him, but did he feel the same about her? I suppose because of the rough start she'd had in life I was very protective of her. However, she was an adult and I needed to have faith in her decisions.

Have you got your overnight things with you? I texted, practical to the last.

Yes. 👍

So this had been planned ahead and she'd taken what she needed with her to work.

I replied: *OK, love. Thanks for letting me know. I look forward to meeting Darren. Love, Mum xxx*

Much later, I wondered if I'd done the right thing, but how wise we are in hindsight! And realistically, would me saying I didn't think spending the night with Darren was a good idea and they should get to know each other better first have made any difference? Probably not.

CHAPTER EIGHTEEN

FAMILY

After all the upset and turmoil of Oskar revealing he had been sexually abused, our lives settled down for a while. May slipped into June and the weather grew warmer. Flowers bloomed, birds sang and everyone looked that bit happier, even Oskar. Of course, it was a huge relief for him, and us, that he had been able to tell, and his abusers were being sought by the police. I asked him again if he would like to invite a friend from school home for tea. He wasn't overly enthusiastic and said quaintly he'd think about it. He liked PE at school and was good at it, so I enrolled him in a Saturday-morning gym class for children at our local sports centre. The session was an hour long and he thoroughly enjoyed it, and it gave him a new interest.

The final court hearing for the child-care proceedings was scheduled for October. If Oskar wasn't returned to his mother (which was unlikely), I assumed he would stay with me. But that was all in the future, and our routine continued with school and the same contact arrangements, the quality of which didn't improve, so that Oskar's relationship with his mother stayed the same – cool. I had hoped that after Roksana's initial upset at learning Oskar had been abused, she might have invested more time in him, but that didn't happen.

Contact remained an hour twice a week and she often arrived preoccupied and anxious about one worry or another – mainly work and money problems. I was sympathetic, but my first concern was Oskar.

Now he was more settled with us, he felt secure enough to begin releasing his anger, which I'd guessed might happen at some point. Since disclosing abuse he hadn't mentioned it again, but I knew it would be brewing inside him. I hoped therapy would help, but we were still waiting for the CAMHS appointment. It began with him being less cooperative and compliant, and saying no when he should have been saying yes to something I'd asked him to do or not do. It was accompanied by a scowl, which made him look cute rather than threatening, although it was becoming irritating. Eventually, at the dinner table one evening, Lucy said, 'What's the opposite of no, Oskar?'

'Yes,' he replied.

'Excellent. You need to use it more often.'

'No!' he scowled, and we had to smile.

My amateur psychology told me the reason he was saying no so much was because he was trying to regain some of the control that had been so brutally ripped from him when he'd been abused. He hadn't been able to stop the abuse by saying no, but now he could control other, smaller things in his life. I couldn't sanction every misdemeanour or rudeness, so I let minor issues go and concentrated on what he had to do – for safety or his general well-being. For example, he didn't have to pack away all his toys at night, but he did have to go to bed and get up at a reasonable time. I praised all his positive behaviour, ignored his minor negative behaviour, and applied strategies like the closed-choice technique when necessary so that ultimately Oskar did as I asked. (Details of the closed choice and other strategies for parenting are in my book *Happy Kids*.)

Miss Jordan told me that Oskar had started 'playing up' at school as she put it. I think it came as a shock to her to see this quiet, withdrawn, timid child suddenly assert himself and become disruptive. She'd been made aware of the abuse, so appreciated why Oskar's behaviour had deteriorated. I assumed she could deal with it – she was, after all, a trained teacher. But then one afternoon she came out looking very worried and said there'd been an incident in the classroom. Apparently, when Oskar had been asked to pack away his art work at the end of the lesson, as the other children were doing, he'd sworn at her and then flown into a rage. He'd kicked over easels and thrown paint around. Miss Jordan had splodges of paint on her blouse.

'That was very naughty,' I told Oskar, who was standing beside us. Then to Miss Jordan I said, 'I hope you sanctioned him.'

'Oh no,' she replied. 'I wouldn't do that. I understand why he's angry, the poor child. I had a little chat with him and hopefully he won't do it again.'

Miss Jordan was a kind, sensitive teacher and naturally felt sorry for Oskar, but having a little chat with him hadn't stopped him playing up before. Indeed, his behaviour at school was worse than it was at home.

'I know it's difficult,' I said. 'But Oskar does need boundaries for good behaviour, just as all the other children do. I am sanctioning him at home when he's done something wrong.'

'Are you?' she asked. I could tell from her expression she thought I was being harsh.

'It's natural for Oskar to feel angry about what happened,' I said, aware he could hear me. 'But he will need to behave himself like the other children in the class do. I'll deal with this, and please let me know if there are further instances. It will help if he sees us working together.'

'Thank you,' she said. Then to Oskar, 'We'll have a better day tomorrow.'

Oskar looked at me apprehensively as we walked away. 'I know you're angry because of what happened,' I said. 'But kicking off at school isn't the way to deal with it. You need to do as your teacher tells you. You've lost fifteen minutes of garden time.'

'Don't care,' he said, pulling a face. But I knew he did care, for now the summer was here he enjoyed going into the garden to play as soon as we arrived home from school.

'I don't like you,' he said as I opened the car door.

'That's a pity because I like you. Lots.'

'Don't care,' he said again. Then as I drove, he said more forcefully, 'I really don't like you. I'm not pretending.'

I stifled a smile. 'OK, but you're still going to do as you're told, and I like you just the same.' I saw him stick out his tongue, which I ignored.

Once home, Oskar sat in the living room gazing forlornly through the window until the fifteen minutes were up and I opened the patio door for him to go out. Yes, I felt like a wicked witch, but putting in place boundaries for good behaviour is a sign of caring, and children have to learn correct behaviour to become well-adjusted, responsible adults. I didn't want what had happened to ruin Oskar's future, which it could easily have done. However, I appreciated it was easier for me, dealing with one child, than for Miss Jordan, who had a classroom full. I was doing all I could to help her, but I had the feeling this was going to get worse before it got better.

Oskar began stealing food again from the other children's packed lunches, although there was no need, as he was being well fed at home by me and always had breakfast. At the same time, he started being cruel to other children – those smaller and more vulnerable than himself – pushing them over and hitting them. While it was very wrong, I could see the logic: as he'd been hurt by his abusers, so he was hurting others. One playtime he threatened a lad that he would cut him up into little pieces and described it in such gory detail that the boy went crying to the playground supervisor, who reported the incident to Miss Jordan. She was now sanctioning Oskar's negative behaviour by loss of playtime, and I always told him off at the end of school if there'd been an incident, although I didn't add another punishment as that would have been excessive.

One afternoon Elaine Summer, the Head Teacher, came to see me as I waited in the playground. I could tell from her expression it was something serious. She took me aside so we couldn't be overheard and said a parent had telephoned the school, complaining about Oskar's behaviour. While her son had been in the toilets, Oskar had gone in and demanded he take off his trousers and bend over so he could see his bottom or he'd cut him into bits. I was appalled, and concerned for the victim, although I knew why Oskar was behaving like this, as did the Head. He was trying to exorcize what had been done to him in the only way he knew now – by repeating it. Children who have been sexually abused often display sexualized behaviour. Elaine said she'd dealt with it and had reassured the parent without breaking confidentiality by giving details of the abuse Oskar had suffered. She'd also spoken to the boy and reassured him as well as talking sternly to Oskar.

'I thought he was supposed to be seeing a therapist,' she added.

'Yes, I'm still waiting for an appointment. I'll phone his social worker when I get home.'

'Please do, and let me know the outcome. I don't want any more instances like this.'

'No, indeed,' I agreed. 'I am sorry.' I felt responsible for Oskar's behaviour, as most parents and carers do if their child misbehaves.

Although the Head had said she'd dealt with the matter and had spoken to Oskar, I wanted to reinforce to him some basic guidelines about the privacy of our bodies, as I'd done with other children. Once home, I settled Oskar at the table in our kitchen-diner with a drink and I took out a large sheet of plain paper and some crayons. I sat beside him and asked him to draw the outline of a person, which he did. I told him to colour in red all the parts of the body that were private, and then those in green that others could see and touch with our permission. It was an exercise I'd used before, and I know schools do similar.

As we worked, we talked about it. Hands and feet were green, as it's all right to hold someone's hand with their permission or see their feet. But the bottom and genitals were red, as were older girls' breasts. Oskar knew which parts of the body were considered private, unlike some children I'd fostered who'd been so badly sexually abused for so long that they didn't think any part of their body was private and theirs to own. We talked about arms and legs and what should be considered private, and decided that from the ankle to the knee wasn't really private but the top of our legs were. I concluded by saying, 'I know those wicked men made you show your private parts, but that was very wrong of them.

You mustn't do it to anyone else because it will hurt them as it hurt you.'

'I know,' Oskar said sadly. 'I felt bad after. I had to say sorry.'

'All right. You know not to do it again.' I'd done as much as I could for now.

While Oskar was playing in the garden – I could see him from the kitchen window – I telephoned Andrew, but it went through to voicemail. I left a message explaining what had happened at school and that the Head felt, as I did, that the sooner Oskar began therapy, the better.

The following day I received an email from Andrew saying he'd spoken to CAMHS and a letter with an appointment for Oskar was in the post. I assumed he'd managed to move him up the waiting list. In the afternoon, when I collected Oskar from school, I went into reception and asked the secretary to tell the Head that an appointment for Oskar to attend CAMHS was on its way.

Later that afternoon I met Lucy's boyfriend, Darren, briefly. Lucy texted to say she didn't need dinner as she was going out with him but they were stopping by first so she could change her clothes. I was in the kitchen preparing our dinner when I heard the front door open. 'Hi!' I called. 'We're in here.' Oskar was with me as it had started to rain, so he'd come in from the garden.

'This is Darren,' Lucy said, coming into the kitchen-diner.

'Lovely to meet you.' I stopped what I was doing.

'And you,' he replied a little self-consciously.

'Would you like a drink?' I asked him.

'No,' Lucy replied on his behalf. 'I won't be long.'

'Have a seat,' I said, gesturing to the table and chairs in the kitchen-diner.

Darren pulled out a chair and sat down as Lucy disappeared up to her bedroom. He was about five feet ten, of average build, with brown hair. He was a bit awkward talking to me but related more easily to Oskar, I guessed from working with children in the nursery.

Lucy got changed incredibly quickly and then he was whisked away. 'Nice meeting you!' I called. 'See you again soon.'

'Yes, thank you.'

Lucy wasn't late back and I was still up. 'Did you have a good evening?' I asked her.

'Yes, thanks.'

'Darren seems very pleasant.'

'Yes, he is.'

'And he treats you well?'

'Oh, Mum! Of course.'

I hugged her goodnight. My family were growing up fast.

We were now halfway through June and with just over a month to go before school broke up for the long summer holidays, I realized I should have booked a holiday by now. It's often difficult for foster carers to plan ahead. We need permission to take the child on holiday, and often can't be sure if we will still have the child at the time of the holiday, or if we'll have a different child, or none at all. But I now knew Oskar would be with me until October at least so I raised the matter of a holiday with my family. Gone were the days when they were little and I could assume they'd all be coming with me. Adrian said he and Kirsty were thinking of going youth hostelling in the Lake District. Paula said she'd come with me and Oskar, and Lucy replied that she and Darren were camping at a four-day music festival and she couldn't take any more time off during the summer. She worked in a private nursery, so unlike schools and colleges it wasn't closed for the long holidays and the employees had standard annual leave, as did Adrian. Now I knew who was coming with me – Paula and Oskar – I emailed Andrew and asked if I could take Oskar on a week's holiday in August, preferably abroad. If I was given permission, I'd immediately start looking for a last-minute package deal. I knew Oskar had a passport, which can be a problem for some children in care. Their social worker has to apply for a copy of their birth certificate before they can apply for a passport, which can take some time.

While I was waiting to hear from Andrew, I telephoned my mother and asked if she'd like to come on holiday with us. I explained it would either be a holiday in this country or a package deal abroad if I had permission to take Oskar. She thanked me but said she was going to spend the summer quietly at home pottering in the garden. I tried to persuade her, but I couldn't change her mind, so I had to respect her decision. Now in her eighties and widowed, she found comfort in being at home surrounded by the familiar, which held many happy memories, although she still enjoyed days out and staying with us for a few nights.

I didn't hear back from Andrew, but the next day at the start of contact Roksana said he'd left a message on her voicemail. 'Something about you taking Oskar on holiday?' she said somewhat confrontationally.

I explained what I was thinking – a package holiday in Europe or a holiday let near the coast in England. I said that my youngest daughter, Paula, would be coming with us and then waited for her reply. The manner in which she'd approached me suggested she was hostile to the idea, which would put a stop to it before the final court hearing in October. After that, assuming the social services were granted a Full Care Order, they could make the decision even if the parent didn't agree. Some parents of children in care are happy to let their children go on holiday with the foster family, others are not, and some refuse simply because they can.

But Roksana replied, 'That will be nice for Oskar. Thank you. He's never been on a holiday before. Neither have I.' Immediately I choked up.

'It's a pity I can't take you too,' I said. 'But it wouldn't be appropriate with the care proceedings on-going.'

'I know, and I have to work. My holidays are going to see Luka.' My heart went out to her. If ever a woman needed and deserved a relaxing break, it was Roksana. She looked permanently worn out and stressed, but I knew she wouldn't be allowed to come on holiday with us. Had we been working towards Oskar returning home then it might have been appropriate, but at present the care plan was that Oskar would remain in foster care. 'Can he phone me while you're away?' she asked.

'Yes, of course.'

'It doesn't have to be every night. A couple of times, just to reassure me.'

'Yes, we will.'

She then turned to Oskar, who'd been standing by us, listening. I hadn't told him I was hoping to take him on holiday as I wanted to obtain permission first. 'Aren't you lucky, going on a summer holiday?' she said to him, and he smiled, bemused.

'I'll need to check with Andrew first,' I said. 'Although I don't think he'll have any objection.' Generally, the social services like children in care to go on holiday with their foster family unless circumstances don't allow it. I said goodbye, that I'd see them at five o'clock, and left the Family Centre.

As I sat in my car with the windows down to let in some air, I called Andrew. 'It's Cathy, Oskar's carer. I emailed you about taking Oskar on holiday.'

'Yes, I'm waiting to hear back from Roksana.'

'I've just seen her at contact and she has no objection; indeed, she is happy for Oskar to have a holiday. Can I go ahead and book something in Europe?'

'I don't see why not. Send me the details as soon as you've booked.'

'I will. I'll need Oskar's passport.'

'Roksana has it.'

'I'll ask her for it then. I'll also need a letter of consent from you.' This was necessary when taking a looked-after child abroad in case the carer was stopped at border control and asked why they were travelling with a child who wasn't their own.

'Will Oskar need additional vaccinations?' Andrew asked.

'I don't think so as it will be in Europe, but I'll check once I know exactly where we're going.'

'OK. Thanks.'

Having said goodbye, I remained in the car, phone in hand, and began googling last-minute holiday packages. I came up with a number of possibilities, which I noted down and would explore more fully when I got home. At five o'clock I returned to the Family Centre. I told Oskar and his mother that Andrew had given permission and I'd try to book a holiday this evening. I asked Roksana for his passport.

'When are you going?' she asked.

'August.'

'Plenty of time then,' she replied.

There was, but I would feel happier once I had Oskar's passport, as I knew other foster carers who'd had their holiday plans scuppered at the eleventh hour because they didn't have the child's passport.

Oskar was talkative in the car going home and asked me about holidays. He knew children at school went on holiday but hadn't been on one himself, so I told him all about holidays and that he'd have a lovely time. After dinner, while Paula played with Oskar in the living room, I sat at the computer in the front room and continued the research I'd begun in the car. I found it so much easier working on a larger screen. Fifteen minutes later I had found what I was looking for. 'How does Crete sound?' I called to Paula and Oskar. 'An all-inclusive beach hotel.'

'Sounds good!' Paula replied, and immediately they appeared. I scrolled through the photos of the resort, swimming pools, beach and local places of interest to show them.

'There is one family room left for the first week in August,' I said. Paula appreciated that, aged six, Oskar would be sleeping in our room.

'Shall I book it then?' I asked.

'Yes, go for it,' Paula said.

'Go for it,' Oskar repeated, smiling.

'OK.'

Paula returned to the living room with Oskar so I could concentrate. I booked the holiday and travel insurance, and then spent a few anxious minutes checking the details, paranoid that I'd pressed the wrong button and booked something completely different. When the confirmatory email came through, I checked that carefully too, and was finally convinced everything was correct. I pre-booked seats on the plane to make sure we were all sitting together. I checked what vaccinations were required, if any, and then sent Andrew all the details, including flight times and the hotel address. I was excited by the prospect of going on holiday, but my thoughts returned to Roksana. Her selfless act had allowed not only her son to go abroad on a nice holiday, but Paula and me too, for I wouldn't have put Oskar in respite care with another foster carer and gone without him. He'd only just built up trust in us, and apart from that, he was one of the family for however long he was with us.

CHAPTER NINETEEN

THERAPY

The following day Oskar told Miss Jordan and one of his friends, Leo, he was going on holiday, and he finally decided he'd like to invite Leo back to play. Straight away I found Leo's mother in the playground, introduced myself and asked her if Leo would like to come to play after school one afternoon and have some dinner with us.

'I'm sure he would,' she said, smiling. 'Leo has talked about Oskar. You must be his aunt. Oskar said he lives with you as his mother has to work.'

'I'm his foster carer actually, so like an aunt,' I replied. Many children in care tell their classmates they are living with an aunt or family friend so they don't have to admit they're in care. But Leo's mother was trusting me with her son, so she had a right to know the situation.

'Oh, OK,' she said easily. That's neat.'

'I expect Oskar felt more comfortable calling me an aunt,' I added.

'Yes, that makes sense. I've seen you in the playground collecting him. My husband and I have talked about fostering when we have a spare bedroom.'

'I'm sure your application would be appreciated. There's always a shortage of foster carers.' We then arranged for Leo to come to play on Friday and swapped contact details. She was called Julia and seemed very pleasant.

Oskar was excited in the car as I drove us home and I was pleased he now felt comfortable enough to invite a friend home – something he'd never done when he'd lived with his mother, which was just as well, as there'd been paedophiles in the house. I shuddered at the thought of who their next victims might be, for as far as I knew they hadn't been caught yet.

That evening Oskar told his mother on the phone Leo was coming to play, and they had something approaching a chatty conversation, as Roksana asked him questions and he replied. On Thursday, when I saw her at contact, I reminded her to let me have Oskar's passport and she said she would bring it next time.

On Friday morning I met Julia in the playground and confirmed I'd collect Leo at the end of school and return him to her just after six o'clock. I asked her what he liked to eat and she said most things, although his favourite was chicken nuggets, chips and beans. I said I'd make that. I also checked he wasn't allergic to anything. As soon as the children had gone into school, I left the playground in a hurry as I had a half day's foster-carer training starting at ten o'clock. Once that finished, I had just enough time to return home before I had to leave to collect Oskar and Leo.

They came out of school together, both very excited, but Oskar's face fell when Leo told me he had been told off in class that afternoon. 'Never mind,' I said brightly as we walked to the school gates. 'I'm sure he didn't mean it and won't do it again.' Which put a stop to that. Perhaps Leo thought I would tell Oskar off, I don't know; children of their age can be so quaint, even devious sometimes. It's all part of learning social interaction skills for later life.

Once in the car, Leo talked confidently about football to Oskar and how he was going to be a professional footballer. Oskar didn't really know much about football but replied that he liked gym and was going to be a professional – then didn't know the correct word. 'Gymnast,' I supplied.

'Yes, gymnast,' he repeated. Which impressed Leo and he listened while Oskar told him about his gym class.

'Wow!' he said. 'I want to be a gymnast too.'

At home I made the boys a drink and a snack and they played in the garden while I made dinner. When it was five o'clock – the time we usually phoned Roksana – I quietly reminded Oskar we should phone his mother.

'No! Don't want to,' he said, suddenly angry. 'I'm playing. I'm not going to phone her.'

'OK, but there's no need to look like that. I'll phone her and explain you have a friend here. I'm sure she'll understand.'

Oskar returned to play with Leo in the garden while I called Roksana. She did understand and was very reasonable about it, but then she usually was if she didn't speak to him. Most parents would have created a fuss or even insisted.

When I returned Leo home that evening, his mother, Julia, thanked me and invited Oskar to play and stay for tea at their house the following week. Oskar was ecstatic. As we came away, he told me, 'I'm the happiest person in the whole world!' It brought a lump to my throat. Now he was relieved of the burden of the dark secret he'd carried, he was free to enjoy his life, although the harm done by the actual abuse would still need addressing and I hoped that therapy would help.

His appointment for CAMHS arrived in the post on Saturday morning and was for the following Wednesday at two o'clock. I explained to Oskar what it was and that he'd have to miss some school on Wednesday afternoons, which he didn't mind. He wasn't so enamoured with school now he was being told off and losing playtime for being naughty. I was trying to help him express his anger and frustration in other ways, as was his teacher. He seemed to be naughtier at school than he was at home, but I'd found that before with children I'd fostered. Apart from saying no, scowling and stamping around sometimes, he hadn't really displayed much anger towards us. He was becoming less wary around Adrian and would sit next to him now, although he was still cautious of Andrew, but then he didn't spend as much time with him as he did Adrian.

When I saw Roksana at contact on Tuesday I let her know that the appointment for CAMHS had come through, and then asked her if she'd remembered to bring Oskar's passport. She hadn't.

'I forgot,' she said, rushed as usual. 'I have so much on my mind. All this stuff with Oskar. I have to see the police again. I'll bring it on Thursday.'

'Thank you.'

On Wednesday I collected Oskar from school at 1.30 p.m., having notified them by email that Oskar would be attending CAMHS on Wednesday afternoons. His appointment was at 2.00 p.m. and we arrived with ten minutes to spare. The therapy was held in a separate wing at our local hospital; I knew where it was from having taken other children there. Because CAMHS is part of our National Health Service (NHS), it's free to the user, providing a service that many wouldn't otherwise be able to afford.

Oskar held my hand tightly as we went in and I gave our names to the receptionist, then he let go as we sat in the brightly decorated waiting room. It's very child-friendly, with collages of birds, butterflies and animals on the walls and plenty of toys and books for all ages of children. Three other children of a similar age to Oskar were waiting with adults. Oskar and I looked at some books and then at two o'clock two women appeared, dressed in smart-casual clothes. One introduced herself as Dr Elizabeth Fernsby and her colleague as Priti Lee.

'We have someone new joining us,' Dr Fernsby said, smiling at us. 'Welcome, Oskar.' The others looked in our direction. 'As usual I will be leading the children's session in the art room and Priti will take the adult support group in another room.'

I put away the books as we all stood. I felt slightly apprehensive, as apparently did Oskar. Although I'd brought children to these sessions before, the format varied, the therapists were new and we appeared to have joined an already established group. He tucked his hand into mine and we all headed down the corridor, following Dr Fernsby. She led the children into the art room to our right. 'See you later,' I told Oskar, kissing his forehead. He glanced back at me wistfully as he went in.

'He'll be fine,' the doctor said, and the door closed.

I followed the other adults in a room a little further along. It was bright, with a large red carpet in the centre where a circle of chairs had been arranged around a low coffee table. On the table was a jug of water, plastic cups and a box of tissues. Tissues seem to be standard in support and therapy sessions, and in my experience they are often needed. It's surprising the emotion that comes bubbling up when taking part in a support group. We sat in a circle and Priti began with basic 'housekeeping' rules, which is usual at the start of most meetings. She told us where the fire exits were, that mobile phones should be on silent, and other people's views needed to be respected and confidentiality maintained. 'What is said in these sessions stays in the room.'

She welcomed me and said that a place for Oskar had become vacant partway through the term because another child had left the group. She then suggested that everyone introduce themselves and say a few words about why they were here. I now learnt that two of the other women, Nora and Zoe, were parents, and Chloe was looking after her nephew, Logan, and found his behaviour very challenging. Logan was nearly eight years old, while she was only twenty-five, with no childcare experience, and admitted she really had no idea what she'd taken on but hadn't wanted him to go into care. When it was my turn, I said I was Oskar's foster carer and he'd been referred to CAMHS to help him come to terms with the abuse he'd suffered. None of the other children had been abused and the adults were very sympathetic and concerned for Oskar.

Priti now went round the group again and asked everyone to give a brief résumé of the week they'd had. 'Positive as well as negative,' she added.

Chloe was eager to go first and unburden herself. She said she'd had a shocking week with Logan, one of the worst, and felt it was due to him having to visit his mother in prison. She said she didn't want him to go, but his social worker insisted he maintain contact with his mother while she served her prison sentence. 'It's all very well for her,' she said. 'She doesn't have to deal with his behaviour after. It's bad on a good day, but he's been off the wall since he saw his mother on Saturday. He's not angry with her but me! For fuck's sake, I wasn't the one dealing drugs!' Her eyes filled and she reached for a tissue.

'I understand,' Priti said sensitively. 'We've talked about Logan's anger before, and how he can't show it to his mother as he only sees her once a month, so he directs it at you. You are there and he feels safe with you.'

'You're an easy target,' Nora added.

'We see it a lot in fostering,' I offered, as Chloe wiped her eyes. 'The child takes out their anger and pain on their carer. It's very upsetting when you are doing the best you can for the child.'

'Too right,' Chloe said.

'My son blames me for everything and his father can't do anything wrong,' Nora said. 'Although he only sees his father a few times a year.' She then said a bit about the week she'd had, which hadn't been too bad.

Zoe went next and I learnt that she felt her daughter's challenging and obsessive behaviour were signs of autism, although the doctor hadn't agreed.

So while the children were expressing themselves through art next door, their parents and carers shared their worries in support-group discussion. The fact that I was a foster carer raised some interest, and Chloe saw many similarities between the position she was in – raising her nephew – and fostering. Inevitably, the subject of when a child leaves came up. 'I've thought about fostering,' Nora said. 'But I couldn't bear to say goodbye.'

'It is difficult,' I agreed. 'My family and I console ourselves that we have done our best to help the child and hope everything works out for them. Of course, we miss them dreadfully, but some children do keep in touch.'

'Will you have to say goodbye to Oskar?' Nora asked, clearly concerned. 'I was watching you in the waiting room and you seem very close. I thought he was your grandson.'

'We are close,' I said, and embarrassingly I felt myself tear up. 'He's like my grandson, and if he can't return to live with his mother then I hope he will stay with us.'

'Do you love him?' Chloe asked.

'Yes.' I took a tissue from the box.

There was a short silence before Chloe said, 'I love Logan. His behaviour is dreadful sometimes, but I couldn't bear to give him up.'

'No, it is painful,' I agreed.

'He will probably be able to stay with me when his mother comes out of prison,' she said.

I nodded, and the discussion then moved on to strategies we were using to deal with negative behaviour.

At the end of the hour's session we left the room a few minutes before the children, so we were in the waiting area ready for when they came out. I thought we all seemed a little bit brighter and lighter now, having shared our worries. When the children appeared, they too were smiling.

'See you all next week,' Dr Fernsby said. 'Goodbye.'

I knew from experience I wouldn't be given any feedback on Oskar's session, although a report would be sent to the child's social worker. I would never question a child about what had taken place in a therapy session, but I was always positive and interested if they offered anything.

As we left the hospital Oskar said, 'I'm making a model aeroplane.'

'Very good.'

'It's going to take me to Luka so I can live with him.' Which I thought was very telling. Oskar hadn't ever said he would like to live with Luka and seemed to have accepted that he only saw him once a year at Christmas. Yet here he was, one session into art therapy, making a plane so he could be with his brother permanently. Art therapy allows a child to express the unconscious thoughts, worries, hopes and feelings they haven't been able to verbalize.

'Would you like to live with Luka then?' I asked lightly.

'Yes, and Mummy. So we can all be together as a family.'

Sadly, I doubted there was any chance of that happening.

The first week in July, Edith, Andrew and Tamara the Guardian all visited, before the summer holidays began. Sometimes in fostering it seems there is a never-ending procession of professionals, and while it's necessary it can be disruptive to family life, especially for younger children. The visits tend to be when the child has just arrived home from school and wants to relax and play. Sometimes they are grumpy and uncooperative, and I feel responsible.

'Not again!' Oskar sighed as I told him of each visit. To him, there was no difference between their roles; they were all social workers who asked him similar questions and looked in his bedroom.

I told all three of them pretty much the same. That Oskar's behaviour was a bit shaky at school, that he liked gym and art therapy, had a special friend Leo, got angry sometimes, was less wary of men and black cars, and was settled with us and looking forward to going on holiday. In that connection, I also told each of them I was still waiting for Roksana to give me Oskar's passport and that she'd promised to bring it to contact a number of times, but hadn't.

'Perhaps she really doesn't want you to take Oskar on holiday,' Edith said unhelpfully.

'Well, it's a bit late for that,' I said, even more worried. 'She was asked before I booked it and she agreed. It's all paid for and he's looking forward to it. He'd be devastated if he didn't go.'

Edith said she'd speak to Andrew when I brought up the subject with Andrew and Tamara at their visits, they said they'd speak to Roksana and make sure she took Oskar's passport to the next contact.

She didn't. She forgot and promised to bring it next time.

School broke up the third week in July. On the last day of term, we gave Miss Jordan a flowering potted plant and a thank-you card. I also made a point of thanking her in person for everything she'd done for Oskar. She said she was sad she wouldn't be his teacher next term but had told him that if he ever needed to talk he could come and find her, and his new teacher was very nice.

Gym classes and art therapy kept to school-term times, so they stopped for the summer, and I still hadn't received Oskar's passport. With ten days before we were supposed to be going on holiday, I was tearing my hair out with worry and thinking that Edith could have been right and Roksana had no intention of letting Oskar come on holiday with me. It was too late for the social services to apply for a replacement passport now. Stressed, I telephoned Andrew again and he said he'd speak to Roksana. When he called back, he said she'd promised she would bring Oskar's passport to the next contact. I also reminded her the evening before when she and Oskar spoke on the phone.

'Sorry,' she said. 'I've got so much to worry about. I promise I'll bring it with me tomorrow.'

Oskar was now aware his holiday rested on his mother giving me the passport – it had been impossible to keep it from him, as he'd been there when she'd apologized for not bringing it. He was anxious too and the following day, as we entered the contact room, the first thing he said was, 'Have you bought it?'

'Oh my god, your passport!' Roksana exclaimed, realizing she'd forgotten it again. My gaze went to a suitcase standing by the sofa. 'Luka's in hospital,' she said. 'I am flying out tonight. I'll tell my friend to give you Oskar's passport. You can go to the house and collect it?'

'Yes,' I said. 'When?'

'Tomorrow. I'll phone her now and tell her.'

CHAPTER TWENTY

FAMILY

Of course I was sorry that Luka was ill, but my priority lay with Oskar and his well-being. When I collected him from contact that afternoon, Roksana made a point of telling me she had called her friend, Anna, and told her where to find Oskar's passport and she would give it to me tomorrow.

'Thank you,' I said, and hoped she was right. What else could I say? She was clearly very worried about Luka.

I wished her a safe flight and Luka a speedy recovery. She said she had phoned for a cab during contact to take her to the airport and it would be arriving soon. She hadn't had a chance to tell Andrew she was leaving and asked me to tell him, and that she'd be back as soon as possible.

We all left the Family Centre together and the cab was waiting. Roksana gave Oskar a quick kiss goodbye on his forehead and then, passing her suitcase to the driver, climbed into the rear of the cab without looking back.

'Luka's ill again,' Oskar said stoically as the cab pulled away.

'I know, love. Hopefully he will be better soon.' I took his hand.

'I wish I could see him,' he said.

'It's difficult. We'll phone your mother as we normally do,' I reassured him.

'Can I talk to Luka?' he asked as he got into the car, brightening at little. 'Like I did when I lived with Mummy.'

'You used to talk to Luka on the phone?' I asked. It was the first I'd heard of it.

'Yes, when Mummy phoned.'

'I'll ask Andrew.' If what Oskar had told me was correct then it was a pity I hadn't been made aware of it sooner, as he could have been phoning his brother all these months. I'd check with Andrew first, but I couldn't think of any reason why the two boys shouldn't be in contact. Indeed, children in care are generally encouraged to maintain contact with their siblings.

Oskar was quiet on the journey home, deep in thought. I reassured him a couple of times that Luka would be better soon and we'd phone his mother tomorrow. Paula must have been looking out for us, as she was waiting in the hall when we arrived. She looked at me hopefully, aware that I was supposed to be bringing Oskar's passport back from contact. I shook my head.

'For goodness' sake! Not again!' she exclaimed, frustrated.

'There's still a chance. I'll explain later,' I said, not wanting to discuss it in front of Oskar.

'Luka's ill,' Oskar said. 'Mummy had to go to him.'

'I'm sorry,' Paula said. 'I hope he's better soon.'

I waited until Oskar had gone into the living room to play and was out of earshot before I explained to Paula that Roksana had forgotten the passport but had promised to leave it with a friend she lived with, and I would collect it tomorrow. 'I can't take Oskar with me, so can you look after him while I go?' I asked her. It wouldn't be appropriate to take

Oskar to his old home. Paula's college had broken up for the summer and as one of my nominated carers she was allowed to look after the child I fostered for short periods.

'Yes, of course,' she said. 'But what will we do if the passport isn't with the friend?' she asked anxiously.

'Cancel the holiday, or Oskar will have to go to another carer on respite, assuming one is available at short notice.'

I felt as bad for Paula as I did for Oskar, for she too would be disappointed at losing her holiday, as indeed I would. We all needed a break. Paula summed it up when she said, 'All this worry could have been so easily avoided if she'd given you the passport when you first asked!'

'I know, love.'

Oskar had a restless night. He still had the occasional nightmare, but this wasn't so much a nightmare as restlessness, where he mumbled in his sleep rather than screaming out in terror. I resettled him twice, tucking his teddy bear, Luka, in beside him, then he slept in late the following morning. Just after nine o'clock he joined Paula for breakfast while I telephoned Andrew from the living room. 'Has Roksana been in touch about going to see Luka?' I asked him.

'No. Although she said last week he was ill. Is she planning on going to see him then?'

'She's already gone,' I said. I then explained she'd left straight after contact and had asked me to tell him.

'How long will she be gone for?'

'She didn't say exactly, only that she'd be back as soon as possible. She was very worried about Luka.'

'I'll try to phone her,' Andrew said. 'Also, I'll have to let the Family Centre know and cancel contact.'

'I was going to keep the phone contact going. Is that OK?'

'Yes.'

'Oskar has asked to talk to Luka when we phone. Apparently, he used to speak to him when he was living with his mother.'

'Yes, that's all right. Oskar talks about Luka at contact. I read it in the contact supervisor's report.'

'I see, I didn't know. Oskar's passport ...' I began.

'Don't tell me you still haven't received it.'

'We haven't, and we fly in just over a week.' Andrew sighed. 'Roksana said she would leave it with a friend at the house so I can collect it tomorrow,' I continued. 'Can I check her address with you?' I read it from the information form I'd received when Oskar had first arrived.

'Yes, that's correct,' Andrew confirmed. 'Let me know how you get on, although I'm not sure what I can do now.'

'Not a lot,' I said, almost resigned to not going.

Roksana hadn't said what time I should go to the house to collect Oskar's passport, and I had no way of contacting Anna. I waited on tenterhooks until eleven o'clock, which seemed a reasonable time to go, and then, leaving Paula looking after Oskar, I set off. Paula knew where I was going but I told Oskar I was just popping out, although he probably guessed where from the conversation I'd had with his mother yesterday at contact. I used the satnav to find the house and parked in the road outside. It was a large three-storey Victorian townhouse, which I knew from Andrew had been converted into multiple-occupancy living. There was only one doorbell and I gave it a long, hard press. I heard it ring inside but no one answered, although music was coming from an open top window, which suggested someone was in. I pressed the bell again and a minute later a tall, heavily built man opened the door.

'Sorry to disturb you. Is Anna in?' I asked. 'I'm Cathy Glass. Roksana told me to come.' I had no idea if my name meant anything to him or if he knew I was fostering Oskar.

'Anna not in,' he said in broken English.

'When will she be in?'

He shrugged. 'She work.'

'When will she finish work?'

He shrugged again. 'Six.'

'Thank you. Can you tell her Cathy Glass will come at six o'clock for Oskar's passport?'

He nodded, although I wondered if he would, or if he had even understood.

Paula and I took Oskar to the park that afternoon to pass the time. He asked me when I was going to his house to collect his passport and I said six o'clock. I prepared dinner, and just before six I left Paula, Adrian and Oskar eating – Lucy was on a late shift at the nursery and would have hers when she returned – and drove to the house again. My heart was pounding as I pressed the doorbell, for realistically, if Anna didn't have Oskar's passport, that would be the end of our holiday. A woman opened the door. 'Anna?' I asked hopefully.

'No.'

'I'm Cathy Glass. Anna is expecting me. I'm Oskar's foster carer. His mother has left his passport with Anna,' I said.

'Wait there,' she said, and pushed the door slightly to.

I waited on the doorstep for what seemed like ages. I could see a threadbare carpet in the hall and hear voices coming from inside. The door suddenly swung open and a different woman appeared. With a passport in her hand! 'Here you are,' she said.

'Oh bless you!' I cried, snatching it. 'Thank you so much.' I could have kissed her.

She smiled. 'You're welcome. I hope you and Oskar have a lovely holiday.'

'Thank you, we will.'

As I walked away, I opened the passport and checked it was Oskar's and still in date. Then I sat in the car and, before pulling away, I phoned our landline. Paula answered. 'Got it!' I cried. 'We're going on holiday!'

'Whoopee!' she yelled. 'Oskar, we're going on holiday!'

I heard him say, 'I'm so happy! Thank you, Cathy.' A lump rose in my throat, and I knew then it had all been worthwhile.

It was only when I pulled up outside my house that I realized we were supposed to have telephoned Roksana. It was now six-forty and we usually called her at five o'clock, which was between her work shifts. However, she wasn't working at present so I guessed we could phone her now.

I entered the house holding up the passport and Oskar rushed to greet me, closely followed by Paula, both smiling and looking relieved.

'I knew Mummy wouldn't forget,' Oskar said.

Clearly, he had more confidence in her than I did. 'We need to phone your mother. I forgot earlier,' I told him.

I thanked Paula for looking after Oskar and she went up to her room while Oskar and I settled on the sofa in the living room. I engaged the speakerphone and then pressed the key for Roksana's number.

'She should still be up,' I said. 'They are two hours ahead. Unless she's very tired from the flight.'

Roksana answered her mobile after a few rings. 'It's Cathy. Sorry we didn't phone earlier.'

'No problem. So now you have Oskar's passport. Anna texted and said you'd collected it.'

'Yes, thank you. Also, I telephoned Andrew this morning like you asked and explained you'd had to leave in a hurry because Luka was ill.'

'He left a message on my voicemail. I'll phone him when I have a return date.'

'How is Luka?' I asked.

'Out of hospital and resting in bed. My sister is so good with him.'

'After Oskar has spoken to you, he'd like to speak to Luka if that is possible. He tells me they used to talk when you phoned.'

'Yes. Dol and her family would like to talk to Oskar too.'

'Is Dol his aunt?' I needed to know who Oskar was talking to, as Andrew had asked me to monitor the phone contact.

'Yes, my sister. Luka lives here with her and her family. They used to be very close to Oskar.'

'They will need to speak in English,' I reminded her.

'I know. They understand.'

'I'll put Oskar on.' I passed the handset to him.

'How are you?' he asked his mother.

'Stressed,' she said. 'There are bills to pay and I'm not earning any money here.'

'Thank you for leaving my passport. I can go on holiday.'

'I wish I could have a holiday,' she lamented. 'I need one. I'll put Luka on, but don't tire him. He only came out of hospital this morning and is in bed.'

There was a short silence and some muffled sounds and then an older boy's voice came on the line. 'Hello, Oskar.'

'Hi, Luka, are you better?'

'A bit, but I have to stay in bed today.'

'What are you doing?'

'Watching television. Saby and Tamy are here.' I could hear children's voices in the background.

'Who are they?' I quietly asked Oskar.

'Our cousins,' he replied. I nodded.

'Tell Saby and Tamy to say hi,' Oskar said to Luka.

'Say hi to Oskar,' Luka repeated. There was a chorus of two young girls calling, 'Hello, Oskar! We miss you!'

'Hello!' Oskar called back, smiling. 'I miss you too.'

'What are you doing?' Luka asked Oskar.

'Talking to you,' Oskar joked.

'No, in the day, silly. Do you go to school?'

'It's the summer holidays.'

'D'oh! I forgot.'

'After I've finished talking to you I'll have to go to bed,' Oskar said.

'I'm already in bed, but I can get up tomorrow.'

So the brothers' conversation continued, light and easy. Although there wasn't a great exchange of information as there tends to be when adults are talking, I could sense their warmth for each other. The smile on Oskar's face emphasized the bond between them. Again, I thought it was a pity we hadn't been phoning Luka before. Oskar seemed to be getting more out of this conversation than he ever did from those with his mother. Saby and Tamy called hi again and then one of them said, 'Daddy is going to talk to you.' So this would be Oskar and Luka's uncle. He came on the phone.

'Hello, Oskar,' he said, his voice deep, with only a slight accent. 'How are you doing?'

'Good,' Oskar replied, grinning.

'Are you behaving yourself?'

'Yes. Most of the time.' He glanced at me and I smiled and nodded.

'Your mother told me what happened to you. If I catch those men, I'll tear their balls off, you can be sure of that.'

Oskar went very quiet and I was about to intervene and say this wasn't appropriate when his uncle added, 'Sorry, lad, I shouldn't have said that, but we are very angry.' I heard a woman's voice and then he said, 'Your aunt wants to speak to you. Goodbye, phone us again soon.'

'I will,' Oskar said. 'Bye, Uncle Ivan.'

Oskar's Aunty Dol now came on the phone with a very bright, 'Hi, Oskar, how are you, love?'

'I'm good, Aunty, thank you.'

'I hear you're going on holiday. Aren't you lucky? Where are you going?'

Oskar looked at me. 'Crete,' I prompted.

'Crete,' he said.

'Wonderful. Do you know where that is?'

'Near Greece,' he said. I'd shown him on the map when I'd booked the holiday.

'Yes, that's right. It's a really beautiful island with lots of sunshine and blue sea. Do you know how long it will take you to get there on the plane?'

'About four hours,' he said, which he also remembered from when I'd told him.

'How exciting. Are you going to swim in the sea like the fishes?'

'Yes,' Oskar said, his face the picture of happiness. 'Cathy has bought me new swimming trunks with pictures of dolphins on.'

'Fantastic. I want some.'

212

'They're for boys!' he laughed. 'You can't wear them!'

As Oskar continued talking to his aunt, I thought what a contrast this conversation was to those he had with his mother. Despite whatever worries Dol had – and I'm sure she had plenty, caring for Luka as well as her own family – she'd put them aside to concentrate on Oskar, which is what his mother should have tried to do. Dol sounded so vibrant and full of life. It was infectious and she passed this on to Oskar, who was sitting upright, animated and smiling as he chatted, not just about the holiday but gym, Leo, school and the activities he did with us. They talked for about fifteen minutes and then Dol said, 'I'd better go now, love. It's past your cousins' bedtime. Can I say a quick hello to Cathy? Is she there?'

'Yes. Bye, Aunty Dol.'

'Bye, Oskar. Take care. Love you.'

'Love you too.'

Oskar passed the handset to me and went off to play. I disengaged the speaker and put the phone to my ear. 'Hello, Dol, Cathy here.'

'Hello. How is Oskar really?' she asked, her voice suddenly serious. 'We're all so worried about him.'

'He's doing all right now,' I reassured her. 'He was very quiet and withdrawn when he first arrived, but now he's been able to tell what happened and is attending art therapy, he's gradually recovering.'

'I am so relieved to hear that. I know Roksana sees him, but it isn't for long and whenever I ask her how he is she says OK. Have they caught the men who abused him?'

'Not as far as I know.'

'I hope they do soon. We were horrified when we found out what they'd been doing, and in his home! No child is safe until they're caught.'

I agreed.

'Anyway, I'd better go. It's Sabiny and Tamary's bedtime,' she said, using her daughter's full names. 'And Luka needs taking to the bathroom and then settling for the night.'

'Doesn't Roksana do that when she's there?' I asked.

Dol gave a small laugh. 'No, she says I'm better at it than she is. But the reason Luka prefers me to do his caring is because he knows me better than her. I've looked after him since he was three.'

'Really? I didn't realize. That's very good of you.' I knew Luka was twelve now.

'I like looking after him,' Dol said. 'Roksana gives me something for his keep, which helps towards our family budget. Ivan works hard but wages are low here. Most of Roksana's money goes towards paying off the debt her ex-husband left her with. Poor woman. Did she tell you she lost her house because of him?'

'No. She didn't. I am sorry.' The long hours she worked now made more sense: she was struggling to repay a debt as well as trying to cover her and her son's current living expenses.

We said goodbye. I was pleased Dol had asked to speak to me. It had given me a better picture of Oskar's extended family.

Each evening after that, in the week leading up to our holiday, when Oskar telephoned his mother he also spoke to all members of his extended family, including his cousins. It was lovely to hear. I noted that they had spoken in my log and at the end of the week – on Friday evening – before we left for our holiday in the morning, I emailed an update to Andrew. Then I packed my log book in my suitcase and for the umpteenth time checked I had our passports, tickets, boarding passes and the letter of consent from Andrew in my hand luggage. I couldn't believe we were actually going away!

CHAPTER TWENTY-ONE

GOOD AND BAD NEWS

Our holiday was everything we'd hoped for. Endless days of warm sunshine, clear blue skies, azure sea, golden sands, delicious food and buckets of the holiday spirit that makes people smile. Having said that, taking a child on holiday is obviously different to adults going away, as children need to be supervised the whole time, and large parts of the day are built around what they want to do. But Paula and I didn't mind. It was a delight to see Oskar so carefree and enjoying himself. Paula, away from her college work, had time to chill on a sunbed too. Not having to cook was a luxury for me. We were all-inclusive, so breakfast, lunch and dinner were provided, buffet-style, in the dining room. All we had to do was arrive and choose what we wanted to eat. There was a fantastic choice and Oskar found plenty he liked and was willing to try new foods, including the local traditional dishes, which were delicious.

The beach was a few minutes' walk away from the hotel, and the hotel had three swimming pools in its grounds, one designed for children with water activities. Oskar couldn't swim – his class would be starting swimming lessons in the new term – so he was wearing armbands at present. Paula and I went in the water with him and as well as having fun we showed him some basic swimming strokes. He didn't mind water splashing on his face and towards the end of the week he was attempting a few strokes unaided as long as we were close by. We spent most of our time either in this pool or at the beach, but one day we went on an organized trip to see more of the island. The tour included historic sites, a church, breath-taking scenery and a traditional market, where we bought presents to take back with us, including ones for Roksana and Luka.

I took plenty of photographs and would give Roksana copies at contact as I had been doing. It's usual for foster carers to give the child's family some photos, but previously Roksana, preoccupied as usual with her worries, had said thank you and tucked them into her bag rather than spending time going through them with Oskar. Hopefully she would show more enthusiasm with these, as they were of his first holiday.

I phoned Adrian and Lucy midweek as well as texting them, and Oskar told them excitedly all about swimming and what a great time he was having. They were pleased for him and interested in what he had to say. As was Luka, Aunty Dol, Uncle Ivan and his cousins when we phoned them. Sadly, his mother's responses were often uninspiring, and she continued to share her problems with him. 'I've just heard that my afternoon shifts have changed. I'll need to sort that out when I get back,' she told him once. Then another time, 'I have to email your social worker and tell him when I'm returning to the UK.'

Oskar didn't want to be reminded of his social worker when on holiday. 'Bye, Mum,' he said, and cut the call.

I wasn't going to phone back as he'd spoken to everyone, but a few minutes later my mobile rang and I was surprised to hear Roksana's voice. She wasn't supposed to have my contact details, then I realized what I'd done – or rather not done. At home I used the landline to call her, which was set permanently to private number. I must have forgotten to do the same with my mobile. Hopefully it wouldn't cause a problem, but I'd need to let Andrew know.

'Can you tell Oskar that his abusers have been caught,' she wanted to tell me.

'Oh, thank you. Good. I'm pleased,' I said.

'So am I.'

'Did you want to speak to Oskar again?'

'No, you can tell him.' And she said goodbye.

'Was that Mummy?' Oskar asked. We were in the hotel room.

'Yes. Those men who abused you have been caught,' I said, and then wished I hadn't.

His face fell and I saw the sadness and pain return to his eyes, which I hadn't seen the whole time we'd been away.

'So there is nothing for you to worry about,' I added quickly, and changed the subject.

Each evening after dinner there was an hour's family entertainment, beginning at eight o'clock. The three of us went and then afterwards returned to our hotel room. There was entertainment later for adults too, but I didn't feel comfortable using the hotel child-minding service and Paula wasn't fussed about seeing the cabaret or going to the disco. Once Oskar was in bed, Paula and I either read or listened to music on our headphones. The room had a king-size bed, which Paula and I slept in, and a single bed in the recess, which Oskar had. There was enough space for another single bed, as the room could sleep four. Oskar changed in the bathroom and slept like a log, as did Paula and I. But all too soon the week came to an end and it was time for us to pack up and return home. Not only had we had a lovely, relaxing time, but I felt it had helped cement our family bond, as holidays can do.

Roksana hadn't telephoned again since the evening I'd inadvertently divulged my mobile number, but on Saturday, as we were waiting at the airport for our flight to be called, she texted: *I have an early flight back on Monday so I'll see Oskar Tuesday.*

I texted a reply: *Thanks for letting me know. Don't forget to tell Andrew.*

Andrew would have to reinstate contact at the Family Centre. If it wasn't possible for Roksana and Oskar to have the same arrangements, she would be offered alternative dates and times. I told Oskar that his mother was returning to the UK on Monday.

'When she's back will I still be able to talk to Aunty Dol?' he asked.

'Hopefully. I'll need to ask your social worker, and find out your aunt's number.' I'd been phoning Roksana's mobile when Oskar had been talking to his aunt and her family.

'Mummy has Aunty Dol's number,' Oskar said eagerly. 'I can get it for you.'

'It's OK. I can ask her once I've spoken to Andrew.'

'Can I talk to my aunt every night?' Oskar persisted.

'Probably not. Remember, you also have to phone your mother and see her at contact,' I said practically. 'I was thinking of once a week if Andrew agrees.'

Oskar pulled a face, suggesting he'd rather phone his aunt than see or phone his mother, which in some ways was understandable. It was a more positive experience for him.

* * *

It was seven o'clock when we finally arrived home, to an almost empty house. It was Saturday evening and Adrian and Lucy had texted to say they were going out and would see us later or in the morning. Sammy was in and ignored us, punishing us for leaving him as cats do.

'Sammy doesn't like me any more,' Oskar said as the cat turned his back on him and sauntered off.

'He's sulking,' I said. 'He'll get over it.'

'He should tell you what's wrong,' Oskar said. 'Like I do.'

I smiled. Whenever Oskar had a sulk, looked gloomy or angry, I told him to tell me what was wrong and I'd see what I could do to make it better.

While Paula made us a drink, I unpacked the essentials from our suitcases and then got Oskar into bed. He was exhausted from travelling and fell asleep almost immediately, cuddling his teddy bear, Luka, who had also come on holiday with us. Paula went to her room to enjoy her own space again and I sat in the living room with a mug of tea and phoned my mother. We chatted for a while about our holiday and what she'd been doing. She'd seen my brother while we'd been away and also a friend, and had spent time gardening. She seemed fine and I said we'd visit her the following weekend.

I then opened the mail. There's nothing like the stack of letters that greets us on returning from holiday to ground us in reality again! The tedious assortment of circulars, bills and appointments seemed to have conspired in my absence, as if to say, *How dare you try to escape from this lot and relax!* Included in the mail was an invitation to Oskar's second review (which was to be held the following week at the council offices, as the school was closed) and the review forms for Oskar and me to complete. I put those to one side with the other letters that needed to be acted on. The rest I shredded and put in the recycling bin.

At nine o'clock it was still light, so I opened the patio doors and stepped outside. The air wasn't as warm as in Crete, but it was still very pleasant. Adrian and Lucy had done a good job of watering the potted plants on the patio and they'd also cut the grass. The bird feeder had been topped up and a couple of finches were having a late supper. Sammy strolled out of the living room and, finally forgiving me for leaving him, rubbed around my legs, purring. Normality had returned.

I waited up for Adrian and Lucy to arrive home. Adrian returned at eleven and we hugged and then sat in the living room and talked until nearly midnight. He was going on his walking holiday in the Lake District with Kirsty the following day. As we talked, a text arrived from Lucy to say she was spending the night at Darren's house and would see us tomorrow.

I texted back, *Thanks for letting me know, love. Look forward to seeing you tomorrow.*

'Has Lucy stayed at Darren's much while I've been away?' I asked Adrian.

'Yes, most nights. His parents have been away too, so they had the house to themselves. She's fine, Mum, don't worry.'

Sunday morning I spent unpacking and washing clothes, while Adrian packed for his holiday. We gave him the gifts we'd brought back, then wished him a happy holiday and waved him off at the door. He was going to collect Kirsty and then drive to the Lakes. Lucy arrived home in time for lunch and hugged and kissed us all, and Paula gave her the present we'd brought her. We talked as we ate. She was interested in

Crete and what we had to say. The music festival she and Darren were going to began on Thursday and lasted four days. It was being held on a country estate about half an hour away. Coaches were being laid on, with various pick-up points, to dissuade people from taking their cars. She was very excited and told us Darren had a tent, small cooking stove and utensils. They both had sleeping bags.

'You will be careful,' I said, aware there was often lots of alcohol and drugs at music festivals.

'Of course, Mum. Trust me. I'm not daft.'

'I know, love. I just worry about you all, and I can't help that.' I wished I could worry less now my children were adults, but as most parents know that is difficult; regardless of how old they are, they're always your little children.

As the afternoon was warm, we spent most of it outside and had dinner there too, pretending we were still on holiday. Adrian texted our Glass WhatsApp group to say he and Kirsty had arrived safely in the Lakes and were going to get something to eat. Lucy, Paula and I texted back to wish them a good time.

Once Oskar was in bed, I finished the last of the unpacking, put away the cases and emailed Andrew. I'd been checking my email while I'd been away so I didn't have to face the same deluge in my inbox as I had with the physical mail. I told Andrew that Oskar had enjoyed the holiday, and Roksana was returning to the UK tomorrow. I said that while we'd been away he'd spoken to his mother most evenings and also his Aunty Dol, Uncle Ivan and cousins Sabiny and Tamary. I said Oskar had asked if he could still call them now that we were home, and I suggested once a week. I also acknowledged receipt of Oskar's review forms and asked if I should bring him with me to the review, as he would have to be there for the whole of the meeting. The first review had been held at school during term time and Miss Jordan had brought him in near the end. I concluded by mentioning that while I'd been away I'd forgotten to set my mobile phone to private number, so Roksana now had my number, although it hadn't caused a problem so far. I didn't expect Andrew to reply today as it was Sunday. We phoned Roksana at five o'clock, but the call went to her voicemail, so Oskar left a short message.

On Monday morning I took him food shopping, then after lunch, while he was playing, I printed a dozen of the nicest holiday photos of Oskar to give to his mother at contact. I then completed my review form and helped Oskar to complete his. I would take the forms with me to the review, rather than post them, to make sure they arrived in time, as the review was on Wednesday. There was now a marked difference in Oskar's replies compared to his first review form, when he'd been scared, unhappy, anxious and harbouring the painful secret of the abuse he'd suffered. Now his replies were far more positive. He circled many more emojis with happy, smiling faces and wrote that he liked seeing his friend Leo, going to the gym and swimming. I said I'd take him swimming during the summer holidays and we could also arrange some play dates with Leo if he wished.

At five o'clock we telephoned Roksana and she answered straight away. Stressed, she told Oskar her plane had been delayed by over five hours and then cancelled, and she'd had to catch another, later flight and was now having to go to work having not had any sleep. Oskar remarked curtly that he was tired too and cut the call.

'That was a bit rude,' I told him. He looked at me sheepishly.

She didn't call back, but Andrew telephoned a few minutes later and I took the handset out of the living room so Oskar couldn't hear me. He began by thanking me for my email and said I should bring Oskar with me for the whole of the review on Wednesday. He then said he'd spoken to Roksana now she was back, and contact had been reinstated at the Family Centre with the same days and times as before – Tuesdays and Thursdays, from 4.00 to 5.00 p.m. He asked me a few questions about the phone contact Oskar had been having with his Aunty Dol and her family, and then said he'd spoken to her when Oskar had first come into care, which I didn't know. He said Dol had phoned him and offered to look after Oskar, rather than have him in care, but Roksana had objected.

'Why?' I asked. Most parents would consider it preferable to have a family member look after their child if they can't.

'Roksana wants Oskar to live in this country,' Andrew replied. 'She believes he will have a better standard of living and education, and more opportunity to do well.'

Andrew continued to say that he didn't see a problem with Oskar phoning his aunt once a week if he wanted to, but that I should monitor the calls, as I was doing when he phoned his mother. I didn't have Dol's telephone number, so Andrew found it in his file and read it out to me. He then began winding up by saying that he'd see Oskar and me at the review on Wednesday. 'Andrew,' I said, before he had a chance to say goodbye, 'Roksana told me that Oskar's abusers have been caught.'

'Yes, that's correct,' he said. 'I don't know when the court case is yet.'

'So they are being held on remand in prison?'

'No. They're out on bail.' Which I'd feared. 'Don't worry,' he added. 'One of the bail conditions is that they mustn't go anywhere near Oskar.' But that didn't make me feel much better.

'Let's hope they stick to the bail conditions then,' I said dryly.

'Was that my social worker on the phone?' Oskar asked as I returned to the living room.

'Yes. How did you know?'

'You always go out of the room when he phones.'

I smiled. 'That's so I don't disturb you. I tell you what you need to know. The good news is that you can phone your Aunty Dol once a week.'

His little face lit up. 'When?'

'We'll start on Saturday, as it's not that long since you last spoke to her.'

'Goodie,' he said.

I could have added: 'And the bad news is that your abusers are out on bail.' But of course I didn't. I wouldn't be telling Oskar that unless he absolutely had to know. He was doing well now, and I didn't want to send him back to those dark days of being scared, withdrawn and anxiously looking over his shoulder for black cars every time we went out – although it wouldn't stop me from checking.

CHAPTER TWENTY-TWO

ADOPTION

Despite cutting short his phone call to his mother, Oskar was looking forward to seeing her again at contact. It had been over two weeks since he'd last seen her. I gave him the envelope containing his holiday photographs to give to her, but I looked after the gift he'd bought until we arrived at the Family Centre. It was a decorative pottery plate with a sea scene and the word Crete painted on it and he'd be upset if it got broken.

Oskar was chatty in the car as I drove to the Family Centre in the way that six-year-olds can be, commenting about a whole series of random topics that to an adult seem unrelated. We arrived promptly at four o'clock.

'You're in Blue Room,' the receptionist told us as we went in. 'But his mother isn't here yet.'

Oskar's face fell. 'Perhaps she's not coming,' he said. He returned to the door and peered hopefully through the glass as I signed us in. A moment later he called, 'She's here! She's getting out of a cab. She's not very late.'

'Good.'

Roksana rushed in. 'I had to pay for a cab as the bus broke down,' she said, fraught. 'They were going to send another bus, but it was taking ages.'

'Oh dear.' I sympathized. 'You are having some bad luck with your travelling at the moment.' Her flight had been delayed and then cancelled, and now the bus had broken down.

'Have you missed me?' she asked Oskar.

'Yes,' he said, and was about to give her the photos when she turned to sign in the Visitors' Book. He waited patiently for her to finish and then presented her with the envelope.

'Some photos of his holiday,' I said.

Roksana opened the envelope, peered in and then said, 'Thanks.' And put them into her bag. 'Which room are we in?'

'Blue,' I said, and gave Oskar the ceramic plate to give to her.

'I've bought you a present from my holiday,' Oskar said, proudly holding it up to her.

For a moment her face brightened, until she unwrapped the gift and saw what it was. 'You shouldn't have wasted your money on this,' she said.

Oskar looked crestfallen.

I appreciated it was a piece of probably mass-produced pottery, which thousands of tourists take home every year, but Oskar had spent a long time choosing it especially for his mother and had paid for it with his own pocket money. I'm sure Roksana had no idea just how hurt he was as she tucked the plate into her shoulder bag and headed off towards Blue Room. We followed. Oskar didn't say anything, but his face said it all.

Sometimes as parents we have to pretend or exaggerate the pleasure we feel when our child gives us something or does something thoughtful. Most parents do this instinctively, but Roksana just didn't seem to get it, possibly because she hadn't spent much time with her children, or maybe it wasn't something her parents had done. We learn so much about parenting from our own parents or those who brought us up.

Having seen Oskar and his mother into the contact room I went for a short walk while contact took place, as I often did. If it was raining, I sat in the car reading or listening to the radio, as it wasn't worth driving home. When I returned Oskar and his mother were ready to leave, as Roksana was going to work.

'See you tomorrow,' I said to her. She frowned, puzzled. 'It's Oskar's second review.'

'Oh, that. I can't go,' she replied. 'I've told Andrew.'

'That's a pity,' I said. She hadn't attended Oskar's first review and the Independent Reviewing Officer had made a point of asking Andrew to consult with Roksana to find a date and time for the next one that would suit her so she could attend. I knew Andrew wouldn't have forgotten to do this. It was too important.

'It's doesn't matter,' she said as we left the room and then went down the corridor together. 'My solicitor will be sent the minutes.'

But that wasn't the point. Going to your child's review, like arriving on time for contact, is taken by the social services as a sign of a caring parent. I am sure Roksana *did* care for Oskar in her own way, but she needed to show it more if she stood any chance of regaining custody of him.

'Can't you change your shift?' I asked her as she signed out.

'Not if I want to keep my job!' she said bluntly, and with a quick goodbye she hurried out of the building.

* * *

That evening I made a few notes about what I wanted to say at Oskar's review and put those with the review forms, ready for the following morning. The review was at 11.00 a.m., and after dinner I said a bit more to Oskar about what to expect. 'It will be like your first review, but it is going to be held in a room at the council offices and not your school,' I explained. 'Instead of Miss Jordan bringing you in at the end, you will be there with me for the whole meeting.'

'Will Miss Jordan be going?' he asked.

'I don't think so. It's the school summer holidays.'

'And my mummy's not going. She has to work. She always has to work,' he grumbled. 'That's why I got left with those horrible men. It was her fault.'

I certainly hadn't told him this or even suggested it. He'd drawn his own conclusion, and in some ways he was right. It wouldn't do him any good, though, growing up thinking badly of his mother – whether he eventually returned to live with her or not.

'It's very difficult for your mother,' I said. 'She has to work long hours. Most of the people who looked after you were nice, weren't they?' He nodded. 'I know those two men weren't, but your mother didn't know that at the time. I'm sure she is very sorry she left you with them.'

'She never says she's sorry,' he said.

'She did at contact when she first found out what had happened, remember? She was very upset.'

He accepted this with a small shrug, but I knew it would have helped him in his journey of recovery if his mother could have been more open and direct with her feelings. As far as I was aware, the matter hadn't been spoken of again between them since it had first come out. Perhaps she thought 'least said, soonest mended', but that is rarely true of abuse. It often needs to be out in the open and talked about as part of the healing process.

That evening, when Oskar said goodnight to Lucy and Paula, he proudly told them he was going to *all* of his review and it was in the council offices and he would be wearing something smart, not his shorts and T-shirt, which is what I'd told him. They were suitably impressed.

Lucy then spent most of the evening sorting out what she was going to take with her to the music festival. They had to be at the pick-up point by nine o'clock on Thursday morning, and as she was working a late shift on Wednesday she wouldn't have much time in the evening to pack. I knew when I saw the heap of clothes strewn across her bed that it wasn't all going to fit in her rucksack, but I thought it best not to comment. However, as the evening wore on her frustration grew until I could hear her stomping around her bedroom. I went up.

'All you need is a mac, your wellington boots, a couple of changes of clothes and your toiletries,' I said. 'You can get by without your hair straighteners and curling tongs for a few days.'

'No, I can't!' she snapped. So I left her to it.

Later, she came downstairs much happier. 'It's sorted,' she said. 'Darren's not taking much, so I'll have some of his ruck-sack space.'

'Excellent,' I said. 'Well done, that man!' She planted a kiss on my cheek, so I knew I was forgiven.

The following morning Oskar was excited to be going to his review and also a little anxious. 'I hope they don't ask me lots of questions,' he said.

'No, they won't,' I reassured him.

'What about the indie officer?' he asked.

It took me a moment to realize he meant the IRO – the Independent Reviewing Officer. 'If he asks you any questions, it's to make sure you are all right. I'll be sitting next to you and I can answer if you don't want to.'

'OK,' Oskar said.

'Wow! You look smart!' Paula exclaimed as she came downstairs. We were at the front door, about to leave.

Oskar grinned, pleased. He was wearing a pale-blue, long-sleeve, open-neck shirt and navy trousers I'd bought him. I like all children I foster to have a few smart outfits as well as plenty of casual clothes. We said goodbye to Paula and that we'd see her around lunchtime. Lucy had already left for work and Adrian was still on holiday with Kirsty.

Oskar was quiet in the car and then held my hand very tightly as we went into the council offices. I reassured him there was nothing to worry about. I signed us in, checked which room we were in and the receptionist gave me an ID card to hang around my neck. Small children didn't need them, but she saw Oskar looking enviously at mine so she gave him one too. 'Thank you,' he beamed.

'You're welcome,' she said. I thanked her too.

He held my hand again as we went upstairs and along the corridor to the meeting room. I knocked on the door and opened it. Into our line of vision came Andrew, seated on the far side of the table with Graham Hitchens, the IRO, next to him, laptop open. It's usual to have the same IRO where possible. As we went fully into the room, we saw another face we recognized: who should be sitting on the other side of the table out of sight from the door but Oskar's teacher, Miss Jordan!

'Miss!' Oskar cried at the top of his voice. Nervousness forgotten, he rushed to her and hugged her for all he was worth.

'That's a warm welcome,' the IRO said.

'Good to see you, Oskar,' Miss Jordan said. 'How are you? You look very well.'

Oskar didn't reply, he was too busy hugging her. 'He's doing very well,' I said. 'How are you?'

'Fine, thanks. Relaxed. I've had a week away.'

'It's nice of you to attend.'

'Elaine couldn't as she's away and I wanted to,' she replied. Given that it was the school summer holiday and Miss Jordan was technically no longer Oskar's teacher, it was generous of her to give up her free time.

'I've been on holiday too, Miss,' Oskar told her, now far more relaxed.

'Did you have a great time?' she asked him. 'I am sure you did.'

He nodded furiously. 'I can swim now. Well, nearly.'

'Fantastic. Your class will be going swimming when you return to school in September,' she said. Oskar sat between her and me, and I handed the review forms to the IRO.

'Thank you,' he said. Then to Oskar, 'Pleased to see you again, Oskar.'

Oskar smiled self-consciously.

The door opened and Tamara Hastings, the Guardian ad Litem, came in and said a general hello.

'Are we expecting anyone else?' the IRO asked, glancing around the table. It was now just after eleven o'clock.

'Elaine Summer, the Head, won't be coming. She's away,' Miss Jordan said. 'I believe she emailed her apology.'

'Yes, I received it, thank you.'

'Edith, my supervising social worker, is away too,' I said.

232

'Yes, I've received her apology,' the IRO confirmed. This is the problem with holding reviews during the school holidays: many people are away.

Turning to Andrew and slightly lowering his voice, the IRO said, 'Will Oskar's mother be attending?'

'No,' Andrew replied.

'Because of work commitments?' he asked.

'Yes. I tried to find a convenient time, but she works double shifts all week.'

The IRO nodded and began typing on his laptop. I saw Oskar and his teacher looking slightly serious and I smiled at them encouragingly.

'Well, Oskar,' the IRO said, looking up, 'this review is about you and it is usual to start the meeting by introducing ourselves. I'll go first. I'm Graham Hitchens, the Independent Reviewing Officer, and I shall be chairing this meeting.'

Andrew went next. 'I'm Andrew Holmes, Oskar's social worker.'

'Cathy Glass, Oskar's foster carer,' I said.

The IRO looked encouragingly at Oskar, sitting on my right.

'I'm Oskar,' I whispered to him and he repeated it.

'Thank you,' the IRO said.

Miss Jordan and Tamara Hastings gave their names and roles and then the IRO looked at Oskar again. 'Thank you for completing your review form. Would you like me to read it out?' He picked it up and opened it.

'No,' Oskar said quietly.

'All right,' the IRO said, glancing through it. 'Perhaps you can tell us how you've been since your last review.'

Oskar shook his head, self-conscious now everyone's attention was on him.

'You are still enjoying school?' he asked, flicking through the pages of the review booklet.

'Yes,' Oskar said.

'Good. And you are going to gym and have a special friend, Leo.'

'Yes. Leo and me play at each other's houses,' Oskar said quietly.

'Excellent,' the IRO said, as the rest of us smiled. Setting the booklet to one side, he said, 'I'll read that later. I heard you tell Miss Jordan you've been on holiday. Where did you go?'

'Crete,' Oskar replied in the same small voice.

'Very nice. Did you swim while you were on holiday?'

Oskar nodded. The IRO could see how self-conscious he had become and, being used to dealing with children, he said, 'Is there anything else you would like to tell this review, or shall I ask Cathy how you are getting on?'

'Cathy,' he replied.

I said Oskar was doing very well but that since his last review he had disclosed abuse (which the IRO would know about) and had begun attending CAMHS. It wasn't appropriate to go into the details of his disclosure at the review unless Oskar wanted to talk about it, which clearly he didn't. As the IRO typed, I talked about Oskar's routine and what he liked to do in his spare time apart from going to gym and playing with Leo. I said his dental and optician's check-ups were up to date and I was keeping a Life Story Book for him.

'And contact is going well?' the IRO asked.

'Yes, and as from this Saturday we shall be phoning Oskar's Aunt Dol and her family once a week too.' I explained how Oskar had been talking to them while we'd been on holiday and that he wanted to maintain phone contact and Andrew had agreed. The IRO nodded as he typed. 'Oskar still hasn't got any photographs of his mother and brother,' I added.

'I'll ask Roksana,' Andrew said, and made a note.

The IRO thanked me and asked Andrew to speak next, followed by Tamara Hastings. Both their reports were short and curtailed to accommodate the fact that Oskar was present. Although Oskar wasn't saying much, he was clearly taking it all in. Andrew said he visited Oskar regularly and gave the date of his last visit and said Oskar was settled in the placement, was making good progress and the care plan remained unchanged, so Oskar would remain in long-term foster care. I assumed with me. Tamara said that although Roksana was still fighting to have Oskar returned to her, she had acknowledged he was being very well looked after in care – far better than she had looked after him. I found her honesty touching and sad.

Miss Jordan spoke next and said that, apart from some instances of negative behaviour when Oskar had become angry in the classroom, she had seen steady improvement in him since his last review. I thought she was being very generous, considering some of his outbursts. She said he was far more confident speaking in group discussion and generally seemed happier all round. She made reference to his end-of-year report, which Andrew, Roksana and I had copies of. Oskar had achieved a good average in his tests. She concluded by saying that, although she wouldn't be his teacher when school resumed in September, she would keep a look-out for him, and he knew if he had any worries he could tell her. Her warmth and concern for Oskar were clear, as was her dedication as a teacher.

The IRO thanked her, praised Oskar for doing well and drew the meeting to a close by setting the date for the next review in November – so after the final court hearing. He thanked us all for coming, especially Oskar, and began to pack away his laptop. Andrew and Tamara put away their notepads as Miss Jordan, Oskar and I stood ready to leave.

'Have you got a moment?' Miss Jordan said quietly to me as we headed for the door. 'Or do you have to rush off? I'd like to talk to you.'

'I have time,' I said. But I wondered what she wanted. I doubted it was to do with school, as that was closed for the summer holidays. Also, she appeared slightly nervous.

She was silent as we left the room and walked to the top of the staircase. Then, as we began down the stairs, with Oskar a few steps in front holding the handrail, she said quietly so only I could hear, 'I've given this a lot of thought and I am going to apply to adopt Oskar.'

CHAPTER TWENTY-THREE

PHOTOGRAPHS

'Oh,' I said, pausing on the stairs, completely thrown by what Erica Jordan had just said. 'I see.'

'Do you think I stand a chance?' she asked intensely.

'Yes, although adoption is quite a complicated process.'

'I know. I've been researching it online. You don't have to be married to adopt or foster.'

'That's true.' We continued down the stairs with Oskar a couple of steps ahead of us, unable to hear our conversation.

'I have savings,' Miss Jordan said. 'And I would cut my hours to part-time. I live with my mother and she would help with Oskar.'

'You've discussed it with her then?'

'Oh yes, at length. She's very much with me. Since my father left us three years ago there's only been the two of us, so it will be good for her too.'

Clearly this wasn't just a passing romantic notion then, but something Miss Jordan had gone into and considered seriously. 'Have you spoken to Oskar's social worker?' I asked. We had arrived at the foot of the staircase and were now in reception.

'Not yet. I wanted to speak to you first to see how best to go about it.'

'Oskar would need to be freed for adoption by the court,' I said. 'Not all children who can't live with their birth parents are suitable for adoption.'

'You mean if they've got strong ties with their birth family?'

'Yes, that's one consideration.'

'He hasn't got a strong bond with his mother and he never sees his father.' Which was true, but I didn't want to get her hopes up. There were many other deciding factors, and a considerable percentage of those who start the process to adopt or foster don't see it through or aren't approved. Also, at present the care plan was that Oskar would remain in long-term foster care if he couldn't return home. There'd been no mention of adoption, which I would have expected by now if it was being considered as an option. But care plans can change.

'What do you think?' Miss Jordan asked as we went to the reception desk to hand in our ID badges.

'I think you need to speak to Andrew,' I replied.

'But do you think I would be suitable?'

'Yes, I think you'd be very good, but talk to Andrew first.'

'Thank you so much,' she said, delighted. 'I'll tell Mum what you've said and then call Andrew.' Oskar was looking at us now.

'And obviously don't mention it,' I said, rolling my eyes towards him.

'Oh no, I wouldn't, not until it was definite. I know the process can take many months, but at least I'm in with a chance.'

I gave a small nod and the three of us left the building. 'Enjoy the rest of your day,' she said to Oskar as we parted.

'Thank you, Miss,' he said. Then, as we walked away, he said to me, 'I really like Miss Jordan. She's nice.'

'Yes, she is,' I agreed.

In my car I turned up the air con and headed for home, mulling over what Miss Jordan had said. Did I think she would make a suitable adoptive mother for Oskar? Yes, she was young, vibrant, slightly naive, but kind and sensitive. Would she stand any chance of being allowed to adopt him? I honestly didn't know. Oskar wasn't free for adoption and Miss Jordan (and her mother) hadn't begun the assessment process to adopt, which is lengthy and in depth. There are many reasons why prospective adopters don't succeed, and if she was approved to adopt then there was the question of whether she would be considered a good match for Oskar. I felt I'd given her the right advice in telling her to speak to Andrew, and also that I'd spoken selflessly, for I assumed that if Oskar wasn't returning to his mother he'd stay with me.

Once home, we ate lunch with Paula and then the three of us went swimming at our local leisure centre. The pool was very busy as it was the school holidays, with children of all ages swimming, diving, laughing, splashing and generally having a good time, although there wasn't supposed to be any deliberate splashing. It was very different from the calm of the pool we'd enjoyed on holiday and Oskar was a bit unsure to begin with, but with Paula and me encouraging him, and with us standing either side of him, he began to swim with his armbands on. We praised him and then encouraged him to take off the armbands as he'd done on holiday, and he managed a few strokes before putting his feet down. I told him we'd come swimming regularly so he could practise and gain confidence in the water.

Once dry and changed, we had drinks in the outdoor café and Oskar had an ice cream. I watched him licking the cone as the ice cream melted, happy and contented – a completely different child to the one who'd arrived introverted, unhappy and too scared to tell what had happened to him. I knew that if he did have to leave us, my family and I would miss him dreadfully. I had to remind myself that fostering is often short term and children do return to their parents or move to an adoptive home. For this reason, many people decide fostering is not for them.

That evening, Lucy did the last of her packing and stood her rucksack and four carrier bags stuffed full of her belongings in the hall, ready for the off the following morning. She explained that Darren was arriving by cab at 8 a.m., which would take them to the coach pick-up point, so she needed to be ready.

'How will you manage all those extra bags?' I asked.

'Oh Mum,' she sighed. 'Those are going in Darren's rucksack. Remember? I told you.'

'I see, so he's not taking anything of his own then?' For I doubted there'd be room.

'He's fine with it,' she said.

'Excellent. And the tent?'

'He's got it, of course.'

The following morning, I made sure I was up and dressed by 7.30 a.m. so I could see Lucy off. I left Oskar and Paula sleeping. There was no need for them to be woken to say goodbye, as Lucy was only going to be away for four days. I was in the living room, gazing through the patio doors on another warm August day, when the front doorbell rang at exactly 8 a.m. I began down the hall to answer it and let Darren in, but Lucy flew downstairs, shouting, 'I've got it, Mum!' She opened the door.

'Are you ready?' Darren asked her. Then seeing me, he said, 'Hello.'

'Hello, love. How are you?'

'Good, thanks.'

Darren came into the hall and Lucy unhooked her jacket from the hallstand and stuffed that into a carrier bag.

'Do you need all this?' he now asked, realizing that the bulging rucksack and carrier bags were all hers. I thought he was being very brave.

'Yes, I do,' she said bluntly. 'You said you had space in your rucksack.'

'A little. OK. But let's sort it out in the taxi or we'll be late.' It was only the second time I'd met Darren, but he struck me as an easy-going and gentle person who was probably good for Lucy.

He picked up her rucksack and a carrier bag and Lucy carried the other carrier bags. 'Bye,' I said.

'Bye, Mum,' she said, and kissed my cheek.

'Bye,' Darren said.

'Have a good time!' I called.

'We will!' they chorused, going down the path.

I waited on the doorstep as they clambered into the taxi, and then I waved as it drew away. I savoured the beautiful summer morning for a few moments and then returned indoors. Lucy would be back on Sunday and Adrian was returning from his walking holiday tomorrow. I liked it when all my family were home, although I appreciated they were young adults now with lives of their own.

A little after 9 a.m., when Oskar and I were having breakfast, I received a text message from Lucy: *On the coach. Love you. xx*

Love you too, lots. Have a great time xx, I replied.

I am sometimes asked if I feel any different towards Lucy, whom I adopted as a child, compared to Adrian and Paula – my birth children. The answer is definitely no. I love them all equally; Lucy couldn't be any more my daughter if she'd been born to me. She's told me she feels the same about me. I appreciate that not all adoptions work out so well, but for Lucy and me it is as though we were destined to be mother and daughter – it just took us a while to find each other. I know Adrian and Paula see her as a true sister. Of course, we have ups and downs, but so does any family. I feel very blessed to have three wonderful children of my own and be allowed to foster many others.

That afternoon Oskar had contact. Roksana arrived at the Family Centre just behind us; the door opened as I was signing the Visitors' Book.

'Hello, Mum,' Oskar said.

Roksana's head was full of other things as usual. 'I didn't have to go to that review,' she said pointedly to me. 'Andrew told me what I needed to know. I'm pleased I didn't ask for more time off work.'

I nodded and passed the pen to her so she could sign in.

'You all right, then?' she asked Oskar, finally acknowledging him. We made our way along the corridor towards the contact room.

'I went swimming yesterday,' he said, which Roksana appeared not to hear, her thoughts still elsewhere.

'Andrew told me you wanted a photograph,' she said to me. 'But I haven't got one. They're all on my phone and it's expensive to print them out.'

'I thought it would be nice for Oskar to have a photo of you and Luka in his bedroom. If you send a photo to my phone, I could print it out,' I suggested. 'You have my phone number.'

'Oh yes. Good idea,' she said. I felt I'd said something right.

I saw them into the contact room, wished them a nice time and left. Roksana must have begun going through the photographs on her phone straight away, I assumed with Oskar helping her choose what to send, for as I walked my phone bleeped every minute or so with a texted photograph. Fifteen minutes later it fell silent and I sat on a park bench and went through them.

Roksana had sent me sixteen photographs in all, not just of her and Luka, but also of Oskar's Aunt Dol, Uncle Ivan and cousins Sabiny and Tamary. It was lovely being able to put faces to their names and I could see the family likeness, especially in Luka. He was an older version of Oskar, but thinner and paler, and because of his disabilities he leant heavily to one side. In some of the photographs he was in a wheelchair. In another he was in bed, I assumed at home, with the whole family grouped around him. Another shot showed him in a hospital bed with just his mother leaning in beside him to take a selfie. She was smiling, but behind her smile I could see the pain in her eyes. Now, more than ever before, I appreciated just how much stress and worry she was under. Heavily in debt, with a sick child back home and working ridiculously long hours to support him and Oskar, whom she wanted a better life for. I'd known all this before, but something in her eyes in that photo, which I guessed had been taken when just she and Luka were alone in a hospital room, seemed to capture the extent of her burden, and my heart went out to her. She was trying to do her best, but the odds were stacked against her.

I decided that, when I got home, I'd print out all the photos and then Oskar could choose a few that I would enlarge and put in frames for his bedroom. The rest we could put in a photograph album to keep them in good condition. I knew how much family photographs meant to children in care and how often they would be looked at and treasured.

When I returned to collect Oskar I thanked Roksana for the photos. 'It's OK,' she said and, calling goodbye, she rushed out of the room to go to work.

'Mummy gets in trouble and loses money if she's late for work,' Oskar told me.

That evening I uploaded the photographs to my computer, where we could view them on the larger screen. Oskar was delighted as I printed them out. He chose one to be enlarged and framed – a group photo of his mother, Luka, him, his aunt, uncle and cousins. There was also a dog in the photo, which he told me was his cousins'.

'Would you like a framed photo of just your mother and Luka as well?' I asked him.

He shook his head. 'They are all my family,' he replied.

The following morning we went into the high street so he could choose a frame for the enlarged photo and also an album for the others. As well as the photographs from his mother, he had plenty I'd taken of his time with us, which were in his Life Story Book. Foster carers are expected to begin a Life Story Book for the child or children they are fostering. It is a record of the child's time with the carer and includes photographs, sometimes video clips stored on a USB and memorabilia – for example, the child's drawings, and merit certificates from school. It's an aide-mémoire, which the child takes with them if they leave to supplement their own memories of their time in care and help make sense of their past.

Once home, I helped Oskar put the enlarged photo into the frame and the smaller photos into the album. He proudly showed them to Paula – the only one in – then positioned the framed photo on a shelf in his bedroom so he could see it from his bed. He put the album under his pillow.

That afternoon I took him swimming and in the evening Adrian returned home from holiday, having first dropped off Kirsty at her home. He looked very well and was tanned from being outside and walking in the Lake District. He'd brought back a gift of a tin of locally made shortbread biscuits. Over a cup of tea he told me of the walks they'd covered and showed me photographs of the beautiful scenery, some with him and Kirsty in the foreground. It looked idyllic and clearly they'd had a lovely time. He then asked me if I'd heard from Lucy since she'd been away, and I said only that she'd texted to say they'd caught the coach.

'So you haven't seen any photos?' he asked, a smile playing on his lips.

'No. Have you?'

'Yes.' He grinned. 'Lucy probably thought you wouldn't approve.'

'What! Show me, please,' I said, immediately concerned.

'OK, but it wasn't me.'

I looked at the photographs on Adrian's phone. The first one was of Lucy in purple shorts and matching belly top, and Darren in shorts, both painted like rainbow fish and drinking beer from plastic cups. In the second, she was on his shoulders with a beer in her hand, swaying to the music. The third showed Darren crawling out of the tent bleary-eyed from the night before. I laughed.

'Remember, you didn't see them from me,' Adrian said, putting away his phone.

'OK.' But there was nothing shocking about the photos, and I thought what a quaint perception my children had of me. They clearly couldn't imagine that I'd partied when younger, probably because they've always seen me in the role of responsible adult. Pity I didn't have photos of some of the events and parties I'd attended, or maybe it wasn't!

Adrian then produced his washing. 'Sorry,' he said. 'There was always a long queue for the washer-dryers in the hostels.'

'No worries. We can do it tomorrow.'

Paula returned home from seeing a friend and was pleased to see Adrian again. I discovered that she too had received photographs from Lucy. 'I've been left out,' I said, pouting and pretending to be offended.

Adrian or Paula must have then texted Lucy, for about ten minutes later a very sedate and posed selfie arrived on my phone: Lucy and Darren fully clothed, no body art, sitting on the grass and smiling demurely into the lens.

Having a nice time, the accompanying text read.

Great. Thanks for sending. Love, Mum, I replied.

Paula, Oskar and I visited my mother on Saturday; Adrian was going on Sunday, and Lucy would come with us the next time we went. We had lunch out and were able to sit in the restaurant garden to eat. Oskar told Mum it was like being on holiday and he was having a fun time, which obviously pleased her. That evening, once home, we phoned his mother and as usual her conversation with Oskar was very limited and, if I'm honest, awkward. She just didn't know how to talk to him. Oskar was looking forward to talking to his Aunty Dol, which he knew he would be doing after. He told his mother he had to go, as he was about to speak to her. Fortunately, she didn't take offence. Indeed, I'm not sure she was even aware of his curtness.

I left the phone on speaker as I keyed in Dol's number.

Andrew had asked me to monitor this phone contact, as I was doing with Oskar's phone calls to his mother. Dol answered. 'It's Cathy,' I said. 'Oskar's carer.'

'Yes, of course. Roksana said you might phone.'

'Is this a good time to talk?' I asked.

'Perfect.'

'How are you all?'

'Very well, thank you. And you?'

'Good. Oskar is sitting beside me, eager to talk, so I'll put him on now.'

'Yes, please.'

'Hello, Aunty Dol,' he said, a smile spreading across his face.

'Hello, love. Are you back from holiday?'

'Yes, but Cathy's taking me swimming, and today we've been to see Nana, her mother, so it's like a holiday.' They began chatting easily and the conversation flowed. After a while Dol said that Ivan was out, but Luka, Sabiny and Tamary were there waiting to talk to him. She put Luka on first and then his cousins took turns. I kept quiet as they all talked, for this was Oskar's phone contact. Now I'd seen their photographs, they were no longer just voices on a phone, but real people I felt I was getting to know.

The children passed the phone backwards and forwards between them for nearly half an hour and then the conversation began to dry up, so I suggested they say goodbye and we'd phone again next Saturday. Dol came back on to say goodbye and thanked me for phoning. She said Ivan would be sorry he missed the call, but he would speak to Oskar next week.

After we'd said goodbye Oskar went quiet and when I asked him what the matter was he said he missed them.

Although he'd only been seeing them once a year, he had spoken to them regularly on the phone when he'd lived with his mother, so their bond was stronger than it might otherwise have been. I suggested he fetch his photograph album so we could look at their pictures. He brought it downstairs and we sat in the living room, looking at their photos and talking about his extended family until he'd brightened up, then he returned the album under his pillow for safe keeping.

On Sunday Paula and I took Oskar swimming again. He was gradually gaining confidence in the water and each time we went he managed to do a few more strokes without his armbands.

That evening Lucy returned home. She'd texted to say she was on her way and when I heard the front door open I went into the hall. 'I'm knackered!' she sighed, staggering in under the weight of her rucksack and bags. 'I need a shower!'

'Is Darren coming in?' I asked.

'No, he has to get home. We are both on an early shift tomorrow.'

'Oh dear. But you had a good time?'

'Too good.'

She disappeared upstairs and a minute later I heard the shower running for ages, then it went very quiet. Wondering if she was all right, I went up and found her fast asleep in bed. She must have been exhausted. I quietly took the two bags of dirty washing downstairs and left her to sleep. The following morning she slept through her alarm, and by the time I woke her she had to rush to work without breakfast.

CHAPTER TWENTY-FOUR

BREAK MY HEART

At the start of the six-week school summer holiday it seems promisingly endless as the lazy days of summer stretch out far ahead. Then suddenly it's all over and time to start thinking about the new term in September. The last week of August slipped by with days out, swimming and another play date with Leo. I also took Oskar shopping for a new school uniform and shoes, as he'd outgrown his present ones. He wasn't looking forward to returning to school, but a lot of children feel that way. I knew that once he was in the routine again he'd be all right, as he enjoyed school.

I hadn't heard any more about the case against Oskar's abusers, but I was aware it could take many months, even a year, before it went to court. I assumed that Andrew would tell me what I needed to know when the time came. He was away on holiday for two weeks at the end of August and beginning of September, but Edith visited at short notice the day before school returned, which didn't please Oskar. I'd already told him we'd make the most of our last day and have an outing, which now had to be shortened. 'I'm not talking to her,' he groaned moodily when the doorbell rang, and went to his room.

Edith completed the first part of her visit without him and then I called him down, as she had to see him during her visit to make sure he was being well looked after. He gave mumbled single-word answers to her questions and then said, 'Are you done?' and, without waiting for a reply, returned to his room. Edith looked a bit put out, but I thought, as a supervising social worker, she should appreciate that children in care sometimes get frustrated by having their lives disrupted. I can remember a time in fostering when there wasn't constant monitoring and carers just got on with it. In many respects it was preferable for the child, as long as the care they were being given was good. Once Edith had left, we had lunch and then, as it was raining, I took him to the cinema, which saved the day.

The first morning back at school is always a wrench, but it was made easier for Oskar by his friendship with Leo, which had been building during the summer holiday. As soon as they saw each other in the playground they ran off to play, while I talked to Leo's mother, Julia, whom I'd got to know better from all the play dates. She was a lovely lady and mentioned again that she and her husband would like to foster when Leo was older, but he could be a handful sometimes. This was a side of Leo I hadn't seen; like many children, he was on his best behaviour in the company of a friend's parent.

At the end of the first day back at school Oskar came out with the rest of his class and his new class teacher, Mrs Williams, followed by Miss Jordan with her new class. She was scanning the playground, apparently looking for me, and then came over. She seemed worried.

'How are you?' I asked. 'Did you have a good summer?' Oskar was standing beside us.

'Yes, but I haven't heard anything,' she replied seriously, and I wondered what she meant. 'What we talked about after his review,' she reminded me, glancing at Oskar.

'Oh yes.'

'I telephoned Andrew like you told me to,' she continued. 'He said he'd need to discuss whether it was a possibility with his manager and probably someone from the permanency team, then get back to me, but he hasn't.'

'Andrew's on holiday,' I said.

'Oh, that explains it,' she said, relieved.

'I'm sure he'll be in touch once he has any news.'

'Yes. I'll tell Mum. She was getting anxious too and thought it was a bad sign.'

She thanked me and went off to talk to another parent, but I wondered if she appreciated just what was involved in any enquiry to adopt, assuming Oskar would be freed for adoption – which, as far as I was aware, was a big assumption.

By the end of the first week of the new term we were firmly back in the old routine and our holiday was just a distant happy memory. Gym club and art therapy resumed, Oskar continued to see his mother at the Family Centre two days a week and phoned her on the other evenings. Sometimes she didn't pick up and he left a message on her voicemail. We called Dol again on Saturday and Oskar spoke to everyone, including Ivan, who told him about the construction site he worked on. I made a short note of all the phone contact in my log as I was supposed to.

The following week swimming lessons began at school and Oskar was a bit apprehensive, as Paula and I wouldn't be there to help him in the water.

'Don't worry, you won't be made to do anything you don't want to,' I reassured him. 'And there will be children there who can't swim at all.' I knew from experience that there was a huge spectrum in children's ability in most subjects and activities at this age, depending on their maturity, the opportunities they'd had and their confidence in tackling new things.

At the end of school Oskar came out with his swimming bag slung over his shoulder, just as Adrian used to. 'So how did it go?' I asked him.

'I'm in the middle group,' he told me proudly. 'Some kids can swim all by themselves, but others are scared of the water and didn't want to go in.'

'You did well then,' I said. We began across the playground.

'Leo wasn't as good as me,' Oskar whispered.

'I'm sure he's good at other things,' I replied.

He thought for a moment and then said, 'Yes, he can run faster than me.'

'There you go then. We can't all be good at everything.'

'Ramesh is,' Oskar replied. 'He's in the top group for swimming, maths and literacy. He has a tutor, and he's learning to play the piano and violin.'

'Would you like to learn a musical instrument?' I asked him.

'Nah. He has to practise two hours a day. An hour in the morning before he comes to school and an hour in the evening. He's not allowed to play outside until he's done his practice.'

* * *

The following Monday Paula returned to college and the September air had a chill in it, warning us that autumn wasn't far away. On Tuesday morning Andrew telephoned and I asked him if he'd had a good holiday. He said he had and then asked for an update on Oskar. 'I believe Erica Jordan has been in touch with you,' I concluded.

'Yes, I need to call her,' he replied, but didn't elaborate. 'Does Oskar talk about his brother, Luka?' he asked.

'Yes, he does now we're phoning regularly.'

'What about Roksana? Does Oskar miss his mother?'

Difficult one, I thought. 'Not as much as some children do. I think Oskar has accepted that she works long hours so he can't see her much.'

'How's contact going?'

'The face-to-face contact seems fine. Oskar doesn't really talk about it, but I assume it's going well. They separate easily at the end.'

'And phone contact?' Andrew asked.

'Not good. They struggle to find something to say and Roksana is always in a rush. The phone contact with Oskar's aunt is better.' I felt disloyal to Roksana for saying this, but Andrew had asked for feedback.

He paused. At this point I thought his questions were regarding the possibility of adoption; that because Oskar didn't have a strong bond with his mother, adoption might be appropriate after all and that Miss Jordan would be considered. But then Andrew said, 'Roksana's sister, Dol, and her husband, Ivan, have put in a formal request to look after Oskar permanently.'

'Oh, I see,' I said, taken aback.

'When she asked before, Roksana was fiercely opposed to Oskar leaving this country, but I've asked her to reconsider.

They will need to be assessed and I am concerned that Oskar has only been seeing them once a year, even though they speak on the phone.'

'There is a bond there,' I said. 'Oskar looks forward to speaking to them. From what I've heard they seem a very caring family, and of course Dol has been bringing up Luka. What's the alternative? That Oskar remains in long-term care?'

'Or adoption. But I'm not sure that is suitable in Oskar's case, especially as there are relatives coming forward.' A caring relative is generally considered to be the next best option for a child if their parents can't look after them. 'I've asked Roksana to think about it and I'll see her at the end of the week. We have the final court hearing in a month, so I'll need to put any changes before the judge quickly. I want to speak to Oskar too and hear his views. I'll visit tomorrow, after school, and please don't discuss it with him before.'

'No. But Oskar goes to CAMHS on Wednesday afternoons,' I reminded him. 'We'll be home by four.'

'OK, I'll come just after four.'

'Will you speak to Erica Jordan? She saw me in the playground. She and her mother are anxiously waiting for news.'

'Yes, it's on my to-do list. I'll see you and Oskar tomorrow then.'

We said goodbye.

So there were now three options for Oskar's long-term care: stay in foster care (hopefully with me); adoption (possibly by Miss Jordan); or going to live with his aunt and uncle permanently. Putting aside my own selfish reasons for wanting Oskar to stay in care and therefore with me, my instinct was that he should go to live with Dol, who from what I could tell was already doing an excellent job looking after Luka, and they were family. However, at present all avenues were open.

When I collected Oskar from school that afternoon Miss Jordan came to see me again in the playground and looked a lot happier. 'Andrew phoned during my lunch hour,' she said quietly, hoping Oskar couldn't hear. 'He said if adoption is considered then I could apply.' I nodded. 'It's the most he can say at present and he'll know more in a week or so.'

As it was Tuesday, I drove straight to the Family Centre. Roksana was early for contact and was already in the room, sitting on the sofa and nervously chewing her bottom lip. She stood when she saw us. 'Has Andrew telephoned you?' she asked.

'Yes.'

'I don't know what to do,' she said anxiously. 'Can I phone you this evening after my shift?'

'Yes, of course. What time?'

'Nine.'

'OK.'

I could see how worried she was and my heart went out to her, although I hoped she'd put on a brave face for Oskar's sake.

It was raining outside, the steady drizzle of a cool, late September day, so while contact took place I sat in my car with the radio on low. My thoughts went to Roksana. What a dreadful position she was in. To be asked to agree to her child being brought up in another country when she would only see him once a year, or object, lose the court battle and have him sent away anyway or remain in care when she would probably see him three or four times a year. If the social services won their case in October – which I was certain they would –

where Oskar lived permanently would be their decision, not Roksana's, although it's preferable to have the parent's agreement.

I felt Roksana was in a no-win situation, but this was about Oskar and what was in his long-term best interests, and to keep him safe and protect him from further abuse. Roksana's neglect had left him vulnerable and resulted in him being sexually abused. Nothing in her lifestyle had changed, so I was certain returning Oskar to her wasn't an option. Tamara, the Guardian, had said at Oskar's review that Roksana now acknowledged Oskar was receiving better care than she had provided. Would that sway her view? It was all so sad. Had Roksana changed her lifestyle by cutting her hours, moving from a multiple-occupancy house to a small flat and putting in place proper child-care arrangements for when she had to work then she would have stood a chance of winning Oskar back.

When I returned to collect Oskar the mood in the room was sombre. The contact supervisor was writing, and Roksana and Oskar were sitting on the sofa in silence; whatever they'd been playing had been packed away. They both stood as I entered, and I thought they looked relieved I was there. Roksana gave Oskar a quick kiss goodbye, then took out her phone to make a call as we left the room.

'Mummy's not happy,' Oskar told me as we returned to my car.

'Oh dear. Did she say why?'

'No. She said she had a lot to worry about and would tell me next time she saw me.'

* * *

I was very apprehensive about Roksana phoning me. Of course, I needn't have agreed. There was nothing in the foster carer handbook that said I had to take a late-evening call from a parent when they weren't supposed to have my contact details, and we weren't working towards her child being returned to her. But to refuse would have been heartless.

At 9.00 p.m. I was in the living room with the door closed, waiting expectantly, my phone on the sofa beside me and Sammy on the other side, although he wasn't supposed to go on the chairs. The daylight outside had faded. It was going earlier now we were halfway through September. I had the main light on, although the curtains were still open. The contents of the room were reflected in the glass of the patio doors. Oskar was in bed, fast asleep, Lucy was out, and Adrian and Paula were in their rooms. The house was quiet and I could feel my apprehension increase as the minutes ticked by. At 9.15, I wondered if Roksana had changed her mind and decided not to call after all, but five minutes later I was jolted to by my phone ringing. Roksana's number showed on the display screen and I answered it.

'Sorry, I've only just left work,' she said, flustered.

'Would you rather talk another time?'

'No. I'm waiting for the bus. There's no one else here.' She paused and took a deep breath. 'You know my sister, Dol, and Ivan want to look after Oskar permanently?' she asked. 'They've put in a formal application.'

'Yes, Andrew told me.'

'I don't know what to do.' She paused and gave a heartfelt sigh. 'I can't sleep for all the worry. My friend Anna says I should continue to fight the case and get Oskar returned to me so we can both stay here. But she doesn't understand. It's not that simple. My solicitor says that the likelihood is Oskar will remain in foster care unless I agree to him going to Dol and Ivan. They have always said they will look after him. I have to work to get out of debt and pay for my sons' upbringing. I brought Oskar here for a better life and I still think he could have that.'

'You mean if he stays in foster care?' I asked.

'Yes. I know I wouldn't see him much, but he will be safe, and have a good education, and access to health care. He will have opportunities that I never had. I know you will look after him.'

'Roksana,' I said, concerned, 'there is no guarantee Oskar would stay with me if he remained in care. I mean, I would be happy to continue to look after him, but he's only six and all my children are young adults. The social services might feel he should be in a family with younger children, or even be adopted. I'm not saying they would, but it's something you should bear in mind. Once they have the Full Care Order, it's unlikely you will have control over where Oskar lives.'

'And all because I left him to visit Luka in hospital!' she said.

This wasn't strictly true, but I didn't point out that Oskar was being neglected and possibly abused for many months before she left him on that occasion.

'If Oskar goes to live with Dol and Ivan, I'll only see him at Christmas like I do Luka. I can't afford to go more often.' I heard her voice catch.

'You wouldn't consider returning home to live if both your sons were there?' I asked.

'I can't. I owe a lot of money because of my ex-husband and they won't leave me alone until I've repaid it all.'

'I'm so sorry. I don't know what to say for the best.'

'What would you do if Oskar was your son and you were in my position?' I was hoping she wouldn't ask me that, although I had thought about it.

'It's difficult,' I said carefully. 'I don't know all the details, but as you have to work very long hours to repay the debt, and Dol and Ivan are already looking after Luka, I think I would agree to Oskar going home to them. Although it would break my heart.'

There was a small silence and then a sob before she said, 'It will break my heart too, and I'm not sure I can do it.'

CHAPTER TWENTY-FIVE

UNSETTLED

The following day, Wednesday, Oskar went to play in his bedroom when we arrived home from art therapy, which meant I could tell Andrew about Roksana's phone call. Andrew said he would be talking to her tomorrow, and also that he'd spoken to the police to ascertain what their position would be in respect of Oskar's evidence if he did go abroad to live. They were reasonably satisfied that the video evidence they already had would be sufficient to use in court, so Oskar wouldn't have to return to give more evidence, which would have been another upheaval and traumatic. Once Andrew and I had finished talking, I fetched Oskar and then asked Andrew if I should leave the room while they spoke.

'No, you can stay,' he said.

Oskar immediately sensed that this was more than his social worker's normal visit and sat beside me on the sofa, watchful and alert.

'How are you, Oskar? Still enjoying swimming and gym?' Andrew asked, trying to put him at ease.

'Yes, thank you,' Oskar replied stiffly.

'And play therapy is going well?'

He nodded.

'What about seeing your mother? I understand you read your school books sometimes in contact.' I assumed this had come from the contact supervisor's report sent to Andrew after each session.

'Yes, if Mummy is busy on her phone or too tired to play.'

'And you're phoning your aunt and uncle regularly again now. How is that going?'

Oskar's face brightened. 'I like talking to Luka, and Saby and Tamy. We have fun.'

'Yes, Cathy tells me you always do a lot of laughing. That's good. And you like talking to your Aunty Dol and Uncle Ivan too?'

'Yes.'

'They've looked after Luka a long time,' Andrew said.

'Because he can't walk and do things for himself,' Oskar replied.

'That's right, and so your mother can work.'

Oskar nodded again.

'I need to ask you something,' Andrew continued in the same engaging and sensitive manner. 'There is no right or wrong answer. I just want to hear what you think, OK?'

'Yes,' Oskar said, but he suddenly looked serious.

'There's nothing to worry about,' I reassured him.

Andrew smiled. 'How would you feel about going to live with Luka, your aunt and uncle and cousins?' he asked. 'Is that something you'd like or not?'

It took a moment for Oskar to appreciate the enormity of the question he was being asked. 'You mean forever?' he said.

'While you are a child, yes. Once you are an adult you can decide where you want to live.'

'I'd like to live with Luka, but Mummy says we have to stay here,' Oskar replied seriously.

'Supposing your mummy stayed here and you went to live with your Aunty Dol and her family? How would you feel about that?'

'Like Luka does?' Oskar clarified.

'Yes.'

'But I'd only see Mummy at Christmas or if I was ill.'

'That might be so,' Andrew replied gently.

Oskar's face fell and his lips moved in anguish as he tried to find a reply. 'I love Luka and Aunty Dol and Uncle Ivan, but I love Mummy too,' he said. My heart went out to him. 'Does Mummy want me to go?' he asked, rejection in his voice.

'She is going to think about it,' Andrew said. 'Think carefully about what is best for you in the future.'

I could see – as Andrew could – that Oskar was becoming increasingly anxious; he was digging his nails into the palms of his hands.

'It's OK,' I told Oskar, touching his arm reassuringly.

'It's not your decision,' Andrew said. 'Your mummy and I are talking about what is best for you, but I wanted to hear what you thought.'

'Does Aunty Dol want me to live with her?' Oskar asked, his voice slight.

'Yes, if that's what all the adults think is best.'

'And I'd only see Mummy at Christmas?'

'Possibly, but you could talk to her on the phone like you do now.'

'Mummy's not very good at talking,' Oskar admitted perceptively. 'She's always busy and worried about lots of things. Perhaps she would be better if she didn't have to worry about me.' I felt a lump rise in my throat.

'Perhaps,' Andrew replied honestly. 'I'm sure she would be relieved to know you were being well looked after. But remember, this isn't your decision. The adults will decide what is best for you.' Andrew appreciated that Oskar was far too young to bear responsibility for the decision that had to be made about his future.

Andrew wound up as he had begun and made light conversation by asking Oskar when he would be seeing Leo again and what they liked to play. He then looked around the house, as he did each visit, and left. It was 5.15.

'Oskar, we need to phone your mother,' I said as I closed the front door. 'She may already be at work, in which case you can leave a message on her voicemail.'

'She's always at work,' he grumbled, his face setting. 'That's why she can't look after me properly. She doesn't love me and I'm not going to phone her ever again!' He stomped off up to his bedroom.

His reaction was only to be expected. The changes he was facing were huge and very unsettling. I gave him a few moments to calm down and then went up to his room. He was lying on his bed, cuddling his teddy bear, Luka, and look-ing very sorry for himself. I sat on the edge of the bed and placed my hand gently on his arm.

'Your mummy does love you,' I said.

'No, she doesn't,' he returned, pushing my hand away.

'She does, very much, although she doesn't always show it.'

'She never shows it,' he said crossly.

'Some people find it easier to show affection than others, but I know your mother loves you. Look how hard she works to try to give you and Luka a better life. She wouldn't do that if she didn't love you both a lot.' I paused. He didn't say anything, but I could see he was listening.

'Unfortunately,' I continued, 'it didn't work out as your mother hoped and bad things happened to you. Now she is having to be very brave and put aside her own hopes and feelings to do what is best for you. It must be very difficult and heart-breaking for her.'

'How do you know?' Oskar asked dubiously.

I made the decision to tell him about his mother's phone call.

'Your mummy telephoned me last night after you were asleep. She needed to talk about what was best for you. She was upset. She wants to keep you with her but knows Aunty Dol will look after you and keep you safe. She said Andrew had asked her to think about you going to live with your aunt and uncle, and she was finding it very difficult and upsetting.'

'She owes a lot of money,' Oskar said. 'That's why she has to work. I heard her on the phone when I lived with her.'

I nodded. 'Yes, I know.'

'When she's paid back all the money will she be able to come and live with Luka and me?' he asked, turning slightly to look at me.

'I don't know. That would be for your mother to decide when the time came.' She was in a lot of debt, so I didn't think it would be soon.

'If I went to live with Luka, would I still see Leo?' Oskar asked.

I smiled. 'I can't say, love. Leo's mummy and your Aunty Dol would need to talk about that. I'm sure you'd be able to phone him sometimes, though, and you'd soon make friends at your new school.'

'Perhaps I could use Aunty Dol's phone to text Leo,' Oskar said, brightening a little. 'A boy in my class texts his dad.'

'It's possible, if Leo's mother and Aunty Dol agree. Now I think we should phone your mother as we are supposed to. If it goes to voicemail, you can leave her a message.'

I offered him my hand and he took it and scrambled off the bed, leaving teddy bear Luka behind. Downstairs we sat side by side on the sofa in the living room. I pressed the speaker button on the handset and then Roksana's number. As I thought, she was at work and the call went through to voicemail.

'Say hi,' I prompted Oskar, which was all he normally said: Hi Mum, it's Oskar, goodbye.

But now he leant forward in earnest towards the handset and said, 'Hello, Mummy. Andrew came to see me today. He told me I might have to live with Aunty Dol. I will miss you if I go, but I know it's because you love me and Luka, and you have to work hard so we can have a better life. Don't be upset. I will still love you. Bye, Mummy.' I swallowed hard as tears filled my eyes. It was straight from his heart and I could imagine the effect his words would have on his mother when she listened to them at the end of her shift.

'That was lovely,' I said, returning the handset to its base. I slipped my arm around him.

He snuggled close and we were quiet for some moments, then he said, 'I should tell Mummy I love her more often, then she will tell me. We don't say it, not like you and Aunty Dol do. I think I'm going to say it more and she will say it back to me.'

'That sounds good,' I said, and held him closer still.

I knew then that if it was decided Oskar wasn't going back to live with Dol but would stay here in care then I would do all I could to keep him with me.

I wondered if Roksana might phone me after she'd listened to Oskar's message, but she didn't. Oskar had a very unsettled night and kept calling out – hardly surprising given all he had on his mind. Each time I heard him I went to his room, reassured him and, once he was asleep, I returned to my bed. The following morning when I woke him, the first thing he said was, 'Am I seeing Mummy today?'

'Yes, the same as usual.'

'So I won't go to live with Aunty Dol and Luka today?'

'No, love. Nothing will change for some months.' I realized this hadn't been made clear to him. 'The judge will make the final decision on where you will live, and the court case isn't for another month. If you are going, Andrew will then have to visit Dol and Ivan first, so you could be here for some time.'

'Oh,' he said, relieved. 'I thought I was going today.'

'No, love.' I hugged him. 'Don't worry. If you are leaving, we'll have plenty of notice.'

However, all the reassurance I'd given Oskar was undermined that afternoon during contact. When I collected him he was very agitated.

'Mummy says I'm definitely going to live with Aunty Dol and Uncle Ivan soon, and I haven't said goodbye to Leo.' I looked at Roksana, who was busy checking her phone. The contact supervisor was at the table, writing.

'Roksana, the court case isn't for another month,' I said. 'Nothing has been decided yet.'

She looked over. 'I've decided,' she said bluntly. 'Oskar will go. I've spoken to my solicitor and he says that's what will happen.'

I felt sure her solicitor wouldn't have been so foolish as to pre-empt the judge's decision and say that. What he'd probably said was that if Roksana agreed with the social services' recommendation that Oskar should go to Dol's then it was likely the judge would rule that way. However, there was the

Guardian ad Litem's report to be considered too – whatever that might hold – and I knew of cases where the judge had ruled against the social services.

Oskar was looking at me anxiously. 'It's OK, I'll explain later,' I said to him. 'Say goodbye to Mummy.'

'Bye, Mummy,' he said, then added, 'I love you.'

But Roksana was too immersed in whatever was worrying her on her phone to pay much attention to him. 'Bye,' she said absently, and then made a call.

Oskar took my hand and we left.

'Am I going to live with Luka?' he asked once we were outside and in the car. 'Mummy says I am.'

'None of us know yet,' I said. 'But if the judge decides you can, you would like that, wouldn't you?'

'Yes, but I'd be sad to say goodbye to Mummy and Leo.'

'I understand, and it's worrying for you not to know.' I'd seen similar before with other children I'd fostered: caught in limbo with their future in the hands of the social services and a judge they'd never met.

As I drove us home, I explained to Oskar a bit about the reports Andrew and Tamara would write and send to the judge, the court case and the judge's decision at the end so he had some grasp of what was involved and the timescale. 'It will be at least a month before we know for definite,' I emphasized. 'Then, if you are moving, it won't be straight away.'

But, of course, all this talk about moving unsettled Oskar even more, and children usually believe what their parents tell them. I found that little I said could reassure him and at dinner he told Adrian, Lucy and Paula he was going to live with Luka. I told them – as well as Oskar – that we wouldn't know for certain until the court case next month, and then afterwards I explained it to my family in more detail.

Oskar had another restless night and then the following afternoon, at the end of school, Miss Jordan came to find me in the playground, looking rather bothered.

'Oskar tells me he's going to live abroad with his aunt and uncle,' she said, concerned. 'I haven't heard anything from Andrew.'

I sighed inwardly. 'Nothing has been decided yet,' I said. 'But it is a possibility. We won't know until the court case next month.'

'I think Andrew should have told me,' she said, affronted, and with good reason.

'Yes, so do I,' I agreed. But at the same time I appreciated that telling her – someone who wasn't directly involved in the case – wouldn't be top of Andrew's hectic work schedule. Miss Jordan had expressed an interest in adopting Oskar, but adoption wasn't being considered at present. 'Next time I speak to Andrew I'll remind him to phone you,' I said.

'Yes, please,' she said a little tersely.

For those who are not familiar with the ruminations of the social services, it can appear illogical, exclusive and divisive. It can also sometimes appear that way to those of us who work within the system. Miss Jordan had made a serious request to adopt Oskar, so why shouldn't she be kept informed?

On Saturday morning I took Oskar to gym club and then in the afternoon we went to see my mother; Lucy and Paula came too. Visiting my mother brought some normality back into our lives. The uncertainty surrounding Oskar wasn't only destabilizing for him, but for my family, as I'm sure it was for Dol's family and Roksana. Needless to say, Oskar told Mum almost immediately that he was leaving. 'I'm going on a plane to live with Luka and Aunty Dol,' he said. I then had to explain to Mum the real situation.

'Oh, so it's possible he'll go,' she said. 'You'll miss him.'

'Yes, if he does go, we will.'

That evening, once home, we telephoned Dol and the first thing Oskar said to her was, 'I'm coming to live with you. Mummy says.'

I heard her hesitation before she replied. 'We're not sure of that yet, are we? Unless you know something I don't?'

'No, we don't,' I said. 'I've explained to Oskar that nothing has been decided, and we won't know until the court case next month.'

'That's right,' Dol said, relieved.

'But Mummy says I am coming,' Oskar persisted.

'It's too early for her to say that,' Dol replied. 'She doesn't know.'

'Can Leo come and see me?' Oskar said with attitude. 'I'm not coming if he can't.'

'Oskar, don't be rude,' I admonished lightly so Dol could hear me.

'Is Leo your friend?' Dol asked.

'Yes!' Oskar replied curtly. 'And I want to see him when I live with you.'

'If you do come to live with us, we can think about how you will keep in touch with Leo. Maybe you could Skype like your mother does with Luka sometimes.' She then changed the subject by asking Oskar about his week at school and gym club. I was impressed with the way Dol had handled it and thought that with two children of her own and bringing up Luka, she was well equipped to deal with Oskar.

We also telephoned Roksana but it went through to voice-mail and Oskar left his usual message: 'Hi, it's Oskar. Bye.' Then he added, 'I love you. Do you love me?' It was very sad.

On Sunday I made the most of the last of the fine weather and took Oskar to an activity park a short car ride away, which he loved. I was still taking plenty of photos and short video clips of him – some for Roksana, some for Oskar's Life Story Book and some for us. It was even more important now to have this visual record, as there was a possibility he could be leaving us. His Life Story Book would go with him and give Dol and her family some idea of the time he'd spent with us.

On Monday morning Tamara, the Guardian, telephoned. Please don't say you want to visit Oskar and unsettle him even more, I thought. She began by asking how he'd been after Andrew had visited and spoken to him. I said he was a bit unsettled but otherwise all right.

'I won't see him again before the court hearing,' she said. 'In your opinion, is Oskar happy about the prospect of living with his aunt and her family?'

'Yes, although he is worried about only seeing his mother once a year and leaving his good friend Leo. I've reassured him as best I can.'

'He probably won't see his mother more than once a year,' Tamara said. 'But then he didn't see much of her while he was living with her here.'

Which made me think the Guardian's report would probably recommend that Oskar went to live with Dol and Ivan, although she didn't actually state that.

CHAPTER TWENTY-SIX

COURT CASE

The following week we didn't hear from or see any professionals connected with the case and Oskar settled down again, so we invited Leo to tea after school. Leo was aware that I was fostering Oskar, as was his mother, but he hadn't considered Oskar might one day leave, until now. Oskar and Leo were playing in the living room while I made dinner when Leo came to find me, looking very worried.

'Oskar says he's going to live in another country with those people in the photograph in his bedroom,' he said.

'His aunt and uncle, yes, it's possible,' I said. 'But we don't know for certain yet.'

'Oskar says when he's living there I can go on a plane to see him, but I don't think my mummy will let me go alone.'

I smiled. 'Don't worry. If Oskar does go, your mother and Oskar's aunt will talk about how you can stay in touch.'

Oskar now came into the kitchen looking a bit sheepish, for he knew this wasn't his decision. 'I bet your mother will let you come,' he told Leo. 'You can ask her when you go home.'

'Yes, I'll ask her. I like going on planes,' Leo said.

When I took Leo home, before either of the boys could say anything, I explained the situation to Julia.

'That makes sense of what Leo has been telling us,' she said. 'What a pity Oskar has to leave. He's settled with you, and the boys get on so well. But I suppose it's better to live with family. Of course we'll stay in touch.'

This delighted both boys and, once home, Oskar told Paula, Lucy and Adrian that he and Leo would still be friends after he left.

However, it wasn't long before Oskar became unsettled again – by his mother. It was at the next contact, and as we went into the room Roksana greeted me with the words, 'Did you know Andrew's with Dol and Ivan now?'

'No, I didn't,' I admitted.

'He's started their assessment. My solicitor said it should speed things up.'

Oskar looked at me accusingly, as if I'd kept this latest information from him.

'How long has Andrew gone for?' I asked her.

'Only a few days. It's to meet my sister and her family and see their house and the school Oskar will be going to.' This was standard practice for those offering a looked-after child a permanent home. But I thought it was a great pity Andrew hadn't told me so I could have prepared Oskar.

'I'm sure Andrew will tell us when he has any news,' I told Oskar. I then said goodbye and left them to have their time together.

So often in fostering the carer isn't kept informed, or the parent knows something before the foster carer, which can place us in an awkward position. I guessed that, wanting to get the assessment underway before the final court hearing, Andrew had arranged his visit at short notice, but I wanted to confirm this and check that Roksana hadn't made a mistake. While I waited in the car, I emailed Andrew from my phone and said that Roksana had told Oskar he was visiting her sister and could he confirm it so I could explain it to Oskar. Five minutes later he replied: 'Yes, I am here. Please tell Oskar.'

When I collected Oskar I said his mother was right and that Andrew was visiting his aunt and uncle, but it didn't mean he would definitely be going to live with them. It was part of the assessment; Andrew needed to make sure they were suitable to look after him permanently.

'They are suitable,' Oskar replied indignantly. 'They look after Luka.' Which I guessed had come from his mother.

It was no surprise that with so much uncertainty surrounding Oskar's future, his behaviour at school deteriorated again. I hadn't seen much of his new form teacher, Mrs Williams, since the term had begun, but that changed now. She came to find me in the playground at the end of school three times the following week to tell me of incidents involving Oskar. While she appreciated the reasons for Oskar's behaviour, she rightly pointed out that he still had to do his school work and behave properly, the same as the other children, and not shout at her angrily when he was asked to do something he didn't want to do. I apologized on each occasion and said I'd talk to him.

'I don't like Mrs Williams,' Oskar moaned as we left the playground after the third instance. 'She said if I'm badly behaved in class again I won't be allowed to go swimming.'

'That seems fair to me,' I said.

'I don't like you either,' he scowled.

'I think you do, really,' I said. 'I like you, so do Adrian, Lucy and Paula.'

He was quiet on the way home, clearly deep in thought, then as I parked outside our house he said quietly, 'I do like you, and Adrian, Lucy and Paula. I'll miss you if I go.'

'I know, love,' I said, turning to look at him. He was so lost, almost as he had been when he'd first arrived. 'We'll miss you too, but if you do go to live with your aunt we'll keep in touch.'

'For always and ever?'

'Yes, if you wish.'

Andrew returned to the UK and emailed to say that he would be observing the next contact and would I tell Oskar. The child's social worker normally observes contact from time to time, and usually before the final court hearing.

'Will he play with me?' Oskar asked when I told him.

'He might,' I said. 'Although he is really there to watch you with your mother.'

'Why?'

'To see how you get along and play together.'

'She doesn't play,' Oskar said, which he'd said before.

Andrew was there at the start and end of the next contact, having stayed for the whole hour. After contact, Oskar told me he had played with him and showed him how to make a paper aeroplane, while his mother had been busy texting on her phone. I knew that wouldn't have given a good impression. She only saw Oskar for two hours a week, and parents are expected to spend the time interacting with their children. But in respect of Andrew's report to the judge and the outcome of the court hearing, it didn't really matter at this stage, as Roksana wasn't fighting to have Oskar returned to her; she had agreed to him living with her sister.

Oskar didn't know the exact date of the court hearing in October, but I did, and so too did his mother. As the days marched steadily towards it, I tried to keep everything as normal as possible, while aware of the momentous life-changing decision that would soon be made. Oskar continued to see his mother twice a week, phone her on the days he didn't see her and also phone Dol on Saturdays. Sensibly, she didn't mention the court case. Oskar went to art therapy on Wednesday, gym on Saturday and, despite playing up at school, he was still allowed to go swimming, although I did stop his television one evening after he'd shouted rudely at Mrs Williams.

The court hearing was originally set for four days but was then reduced to two. Because Roksana was no longer contesting the case, it would be much shorter. It was held on the Monday and Tuesday of the second week in October and the judge was due to give her ruling on Wednesday morning. Roksana had taken the time off work to attend the hearing, and contact on Tuesday was cancelled. I took Oskar to school on Wednesday morning as usual and then had a nail-biting wait before Andrew telephoned at midday.

'The judge has agreed that Oskar can live with his aunt and uncle,' he said.

I wasn't surprised. What was more of a shock was the timescale. I'd assumed it would take months to complete the assessments and arrange the move, and Oskar would be with us for Christmas and some of the following year. However, Andrew said he was aiming to move Oskar in November. The fact that Dol and Ivan were already doing a good job of looking after Luka helped. The police checks had been applied for, the local school had a place for Oskar, he already had a passport and Andrew was liaising with the child services out there.

'Oh,' I said.

'I'll come to see you this afternoon at five o'clock to tell Oskar.'

* * *

I knew that social workers often liked to be the ones to impart important news like this to the child, so when I collected Oskar from school that afternoon I hid my feelings and simply said, 'Andrew is coming to see us at five o'clock.'

'Again,' he grumbled. 'I want to play.'

'You can play before he arrives,' I said.

'I've got homework to do.'

'OK. We'll do that first.'

'No, I want to play.'

I didn't respond to Oskar's awkwardness. I knew the reason for it and we continued to my car.

'You're quiet,' he remarked after some minutes as I drove.

'Am I?' I asked, glancing at him in the rear-view mirror.

'Yes. Not like you are normally. You usually talk a lot' – said with a cheeky grin. I returned his smile in the mirror. He'd come on so much since he'd first arrived, silent, withdrawn and scared. Now he had character, a personality with likes, dislikes and the adorable cheekiness of a six-year-old. We'd grown very close during our time together and I knew I was going to miss him dreadfully, although I did believe that him going to live with his brother, aunt and uncle was the right decision.

Once home, I made Oskar a drink and a snack and then I helped him with his homework.

'Mrs Williams said I had a good day,' he told me as he worked.

'Excellent,' I said. 'Well done. I am pleased.'

'So was Mrs Williams. She kept saying she was pleased, and then gave me extra golden time. Leo said it wasn't fair, as he always behaves himself but doesn't get extra golden time.'

After Oskar had finished his homework, he went into the living room to play while I began preparing dinner so we could eat once Andrew had gone. Paula came home and I told her Andrew was coming and what the outcome of the court case had been.

'Oh, so Oskar is definitely leaving?'

'Yes. I'm afraid so.'

You might think that after fostering for so many years we would all be used to children leaving, but it still hurt. I liken it to a mini bereavement.

'I guess it's best for him,' Paula said bravely, and went to play with him.

Andrew didn't arrive until 5.30 p.m., by which time Paula was in her bedroom and Oskar was watching some television. 'Sorry I'm late,' he said as he came in. 'We had an emergency. I won't stay for long.'

I led the way down the hall and into the living room.

'Hi, Oskar,' Andrew said brightly. I switched off the television.

'Hey, I was watching that!' Oskar snapped.

'You can have it on again when Andrew's gone,' I replied.

'I've got something important to tell you,' Andrew said, and he drew up an easy chair so he was facing Oskar. I assumed he wanted me to stay, so I sat on the sofa.

'What is it?' Oskar asked brusquely, annoyed he couldn't watch television. I frowned so he could see I was displeased.

'Today I went to court to see the judge about where you should live permanently,' Andrew began. He had Oskar's full attention now. He looked at him, wide-eyed. 'The judge has given it a lot of thought and has decided that you can live with Luka, your aunt, uncle and cousins.'

I watched Oskar's face go through a range of emotions: delight, happiness, doubt and sadness. 'But I'll only see Mummy at Christmas,' he said.

'Your mummy told the judge she is hoping to visit you and Luka more often, maybe two or three times a year. And, of course, you'll speak to her on the phone as well.'

'Can Cathy phone me too?' Oskar asked, glancing at me.

'Yes, I'm sure she will stay in touch,' Andrew replied.

'I will,' I said.

'And Leo?' Oskar asked.

Andrew looked puzzled. 'Oskar's best friend,' I reminded him. 'Leo's mother said she'd like the boys to stay in touch.'

'Good,' Andrew said, then to Oskar, 'Do you have any questions?'

'When am I going?'

'We're not sure of the exact date yet, but probably the middle to end of November.'

'So that's about four to six weeks away,' I told Oskar.

His face became serious again. 'Is that when I have to leave here?'

'Yes,' I said. It was a lot for him to take in.

'Between now and the move you are going to phone your aunty more often,' Andrew said. 'I believe it's once a week at present.' He looked at me.

'Yes, on a Saturday evening.'

'So I suggest keeping Saturday, and adding Sunday and then mid-week, say Wednesday. You will still see your mother on Tuesdays and Thursdays but won't phone her any more until after the move.'

I knew this was to strengthen the bond between Oskar and his permanent family ahead of the move and to weaken it with his mother.

'Shall we Skype Dol?' I suggested to Andrew. 'Then they will be able to see each other as they talk.'

'Yes, I don't see why not, but clear it with Dol and Ivan first.'

'I will.' I reached for a pen and paper to make a note of this, as well as the days we were to phone them.

'Any more questions?' Andrew asked Oskar.

He shook his head.

'If you think of anything, you can ask Cathy, OK?'

He nodded.

Andrew then said goodbye and stood to leave. This wasn't his normal six-weekly visit; he'd just come to tell Oskar the outcome of the court case. As I went with him to the front door, I checked that we weren't to phone his mother this evening – Wednesday.

'That's right,' Andrew said. 'The new arrangements start from now. I'll speak to Roksana and Dol.'

'Could you also tell Miss Jordan the outcome of the court case, please? I know she and her mother are waiting for any news.'

'Yes, I will, first thing tomorrow.'

'Thank you.' We said goodbye.

Adrian came home from work and I told him the outcome of the court case. His reaction was much the same as Paula's – that we would miss Oskar, but it was best for him. 'A new start,' he said.

However, when Lucy arrived home and I told her, she snapped at me. 'I've just got in. I'm tired and I've had a shit awful day. I'm going to my room to lie down.'

Bad timing, Cathy, I told myself, and left her to have a rest. But she was very quiet over dinner.

'Are you OK?' I asked her.

'I don't have to talk, do I?' she asked tetchily.

'Bad mood bear,' Adrian quipped. Normally Lucy would have laughed or said something back, but instead she left the table and returned to her bedroom.

'Whoops, sorry,' Adrian said.

'It's not your fault. She's had a rough day.'

I quickly finished my dinner and went up to see Lucy. She was lying on her bed, staring into space. 'What's the matter, love? Anything I can help with?'

'Not really.'

'Is it a problem at work?'

'No.'

'With Darren?'

'Yes, but I don't want to talk about it now.'

'OK. You know where I am if you need me,' I said.

Respecting her privacy and need for some time alone, I came out and closed the door. So it was a boyfriend problem. I wondered if they'd split up, but I felt sure if Lucy needed to talk she would do so, when she was ready and in her own time.

CHAPTER TWENTY-SEVEN

RETIRING?

The following morning we fell into our week-day routine. Lucy seemed to have recovered from her worries of the evening before, although she hadn't told me what the matter was. I'd heard her talking quietly on her phone when I'd gone to bed, so perhaps she and Darren had had a quarrel and then made up. Oskar and I called goodbye and left for school. I was planning on telling Leo's mother the outcome of the court case when I saw her in the playground. However, Oskar beat me to it. As soon as he spotted Leo he rushed over and said, 'I'm going to live with my brother, so you can come on a plane to see me.'

I told Julia of the judge's decision, the timescale and that Oskar's social worker was happy for the boys to keep in touch if she and Oskar's aunt could organize it between themselves. 'Is it all right if I give your mobile number to Dol?' I asked her.

'Yes, of course. Leo's already told me he has to phone and text.'

I smiled. 'And once I know the date when he'll be going I shall be giving him a little leaving party, which I hope you and your family will come to.'

'Oh, thank you, but that will be sad, having to say goodbye.'

'Yes, although it's important for Oskar his stay with us ends on a happy note,' I said, trying to stay positive.

Oskar had contact that evening and for the first time in ages Roksana put down her phone as we entered the room and hugged her son. He seemed as surprised by her sudden display of affection as I was. I guessed the reality – that he was leaving – had finally hit home, although we still had at least a month before he went. I said goodbye and left.

When I returned to collect Oskar, instead of rushing off, Roksana hugged him again. Indeed, she didn't want to let him go.

'I hope I've done the right thing,' she said to me. I assumed she meant in agreeing to Oskar going to live with her sister.

'Yes, I think you have,' I said.

After a moment she straightened and, kissing Oskar's forehead, said, 'Bye. See you Tuesday.'

She waited in the contact room while we left. I glanced back and saw her take a tissue from the box on the table and wipe her eyes. I think Roksana was someone who struggled to show her feelings and felt a lot more than she ever let on. At that moment, with her guard down, she seemed very fragile and alone. Oskar would be leaving to start a new life soon with his extended family, but from what I knew of Roksana's life, it was all work. I supposed she had some friends, and she lived in a multi-occupancy house, so she shouldn't be lonely. But in quiet moments, when she had time to reflect, I was sure she'd miss Oskar and have regrets. He had been the main reason for her living here – to give him a better life – and soon he'd be gone. I wondered if, in time, she would follow him and return home too.

* * *

On Thursday afternoon Mrs Williams came to find me in the playground. 'Oskar's had a very unsettled day,' she said. 'I stopped some of his golden time – that's when the children are allowed to choose an activity.'

I nodded sombrely.

'I'm aware of all the changes he's facing,' she continued. 'But it wouldn't be doing Oskar any favours if I allowed his school work and behaviour to deteriorate.'

'No, indeed,' I said. 'I am sorry.'

'I'll have a better day tomorrow, Miss,' Oskar chirped.

'Let's hope so,' Mrs Williams replied dryly, and returned into the school.

I was about to leave when Miss Jordan appeared at my side. 'Andrew telephoned. He's told me,' she said. I hoped she wouldn't start to cry.

'I'm sorry it didn't work out for you and your mother,' I said, and lightly touched her arm.

'No, it's OK. I understand,' she replied, and seemed quite upbeat. 'Andrew has suggested my mother and I look into fostering. We're going to the next introductory meeting.'

'Wonderful,' I said. 'I am pleased. I'm sure you'll be great.'

'Thanks. I would never have thought about fostering before I met you and Oskar. Mum's excited too. We know we both have to be assessed, but if we go ahead and are accepted we could be fostering in six months.'

'Fantastic. Well done.'

On Saturday Oskar and I made our first Skype call to Dol. I texted her first to make sure it was convenient, and then we used my computer in the front room for its larger screen. Oskar was familiar with Skype, as his mother sometimes used the app on her phone when she called her sister. Dol answered the call so appeared on camera first. She was standing in her kitchen, back to the sink and smiling as she said hello. Although I'd seen photographs of her and had spoken to her on the phone, now I could see her in real time she came alive, and her warm personality was immediately obvious. I began by asking how she and her family were and she asked after my family, much as we did when I phoned. Then I moved to one side so Oskar could take centre stage and talk to her.

'Hello, Aunty Dol!' he said, smiling and waving. 'Your hair looks different.'

She laughed. 'It needs a good cut, but it's finding the time.' I knew how she felt!

'I'm definitely coming to live with you,' Oskar told her, delighted.

'I know, love, we're all looking forward to having you here. Your uncle is making some changes upstairs so you will have your own room.'

'I can sleep in Luka's room like I do at Christmas,' Oskar said.

'No. That's all right for a few days, but we disturb you when we have to see to him at night. Don't you worry. Ivan's got it all planned. Here's Luka come to talk to you.'

She turned the phone so the camera was facing the door and Luka appeared in his wheelchair. It was old and its well-worn wheels grated over the flagstones of the kitchen floor. Dol passed the phone to him and she disappeared from view. I stayed where I was – to one side of the monitor – so I could see Luka. The boys fell into conversation, chatting and laughing as if they were in the same room. The joy and advantage of this type of technology! I thought. Oskar made Luka laugh loudly by putting his face close to the camera, and then Luka did the same. Suddenly the screen was filled with Luka's open mouth and Oskar nearly fell off his chair laughing. I laughed too. A dog barked out of sight and then bounded into view and leapt straight onto Luka's lap, his rear end towards the camera.

'I can see up his bottom!' Oskar cried, and laughed hysterically.

Luka then put the phone close to the dog's face and its large wet nostrils filled our screen. The dog licked the phone and smeared our view with slobber.

'Yuk!' Oskar cried as Luka wiped it off and the boys laughed again. Paula, who'd been in the hall on her way to the kitchen, came in to see what was going on.

'Who's that?' Luka asked as she came into our camera's line of sight.

'This is Paula, Cathy's daughter,' Oskar said, introducing her. 'She's like my sister, so is Lucy.' Immediately I choked up.

'Hello,' Luka said. 'How are you?'

'Good, thanks. Nice to meet you. How are you?'

'I live with my cousins, Saby and Tamy,' Luka told her. 'They are like sisters to me. Here they come to talk to Oskar.'

The girls appeared, vying with each other to get their faces on screen. Paula waved and said hello and then left Oskar to speak to them. As they chatted and laughed, I felt we were like one big extended family. As well as seeing them, we could also see some of the rooms in their house in the background as they moved around the downstairs, which was good for Oskar as it helped familiarize him with his new home. It was over ten months since he'd last been there. From what I could see, the house was plain, with basic furniture and no frills. I knew from what Andrew and Roksana had told me they lived quite frugally and there wasn't anything left over after all the bills were paid. Roksana sent money for Luka's keep but couldn't help further as she was paying off a big debt.

The phone eventually found its way to Ivan, and Oskar asked if he could show him the work he was doing upstairs.

'Not until it's finished,' he said. 'But I'll show you my workshop.' He took us out through the back door, across a yard, and into what looked like an old cowshed. 'This place used to be a farm,' he said for my benefit. 'But all the animals went years ago.' I nodded.

The shed was crammed full of pieces of wood of different shapes and sizes. 'That's going to be part of the new wall for Oskar's bedroom,' he said, pointing to a large sheet of plywood supported on a wooden frame. 'I'm taking a piece off the main bedroom,' he told Oskar. 'Don't worry, it will have its own door.'

I thought how kind it was of him to go to all this trouble when he already worked long hours on a construction site.

We went outside again and as we returned to the house we could see other outbuildings from when the place had been a working farm, but they were all in a state of disrepair now. I wondered how Luka managed to get around in his wheelchair on the uneven gravel and mud surfaces of the yard.

Indoors, Ivan passed the phone back to Luka and the boys talked some more. Luka was now in the living room where a log fire burned in a stone hearth. After an hour, Dol told Luka to say goodnight as it was his and his cousin's bedtime.

'We're two hours ahead of you,' she reminded us, and we all said goodbye. Before I cut the call, I asked Dol if it was all right for us to Skype tomorrow as Andrew had suggested.

'Yes, of course, but we may have to limit the one on Wednesday as it's a school day.'

'Agreed,' I said.

As I closed Skype, I thought Oskar was the happiest I'd seen him. 'You've got a lovely family,' I said.

'I love them,' he declared. But then his face fell. 'I love Mummy too. I wish she could come with me.'

'I know. You'll miss her, but you'll be able to phone her.' It was the only comfort I could offer him. I knew that in the weeks to follow, before he left, he was going to struggle, looking forward to living with his brother, while worrying about leaving his mother behind. I would keep him busy, stay positive and reassure him as best I could. Although Andrew had said he was aiming to move Oskar in the middle to end of November, I knew from experience that delays happened, and it was very unsettling for the child and their family.

The first week in November the temperature dropped and the weather turned cold as a bitter north-easterly wind blew. Edith visited for one of her scheduled meetings. She didn't stay long as she was running late and had another meeting straight after. We discussed how Oskar was coping and what I was doing to smooth his transition home. She mentioned some foster training for the following year she thought I could facilitate. I agreed in principle but pointed out that it would depend on who I was fostering. If it was a baby with contact every day, I'd be pushed to fulfil my own training obligations, let alone spend days planning and giving training. She put my name down anyway, checked and signed my log notes, then, with a quick look around the house, said she'd see me at Oskar's review the following week, and left. As always, I couldn't help but compare Edith with my previous SSW, Jill, and there was no comparison! Supervising social workers vary in their passion for their work, and whereas Jill was one of the best, Edith was only adequate. I sometimes felt her heart wasn't really in it, as Jill's had been.

The forms for Oskar's third review arrived. The review was scheduled for Monday at two o'clock at his school. I filled in my form straight away while I had the chance, stating how much progress Oskar had made during his stay with us and what a lovely boy he was to look after, although he sometimes showed his frustration through angry outbursts, which was understandable. That evening I sat with Oskar as he filled in his form to help him with his spelling of some of the words. His replies were a predictable mixture of happy, sad and angry. He said he wanted to live with his brother and mother, although he knew that wasn't possible.

Friday, 5 November, was Bonfire Night, so Paula and I took Oskar to a firework display at his school. Adrian and Lucy were out at displays with their partners. It was held on the playing field at the side of Oskar's school, and as well as the fireworks and a roaring bonfire, there was food and drink. Leo wasn't at the display, but many of Oskar's classmates were, and every so often a child appeared out of the dark with a parent to say hi to Oskar. He was far more sociable now than he was when he'd first arrived, and I felt sure he'd make friends at his new school once he'd brushed up on the language. I'd mentioned this to Dol when we'd Skyped, for I'd only ever heard Oskar speak English. They were all bilingual and Dol didn't see a problem. She felt sure that once Oskar was living with them and attending school he'd soon become fluent again in the language he'd learnt as a younger child. She now sometimes switched between languages when they talked on the phone to get him used to it, which put me to shame, as I'm not fluent in any second language.

* * *

The Head Teacher's office was used for the review on Monday afternoon, as their meeting room was already in use. The Head attended, as did Mrs Williams, Edith, Andrew and the Guardian. Roksana and the art therapist from CAMHS sent their apologies. Graham Hitchens was again the IRO. Mrs Williams asked if she could give her report first so she could return to her class, and he agreed. In essence she said that Oskar continued to make reasonably good progress academically, although his learning was suffering because he was unsettled by the forthcoming move. She asked if a moving date had been set yet and Andrew replied it hadn't, but he'd inform the school as soon as it was decided. Mrs Williams confirmed Oskar was still a good average, participated in group discussion and had made more friends. She finished by wishing him well for the future and said the class would make him a leaving card with their photographs in it to remember them by. The IRO thanked her and she then left to return to her class.

Elaine Summer said a few words, more or less reiterating what Mrs Williams had said – that Oskar had made steady progress during his time in the school and continued to do so, considering all that was going on in his private life. She said that now the decision had been made about where Oskar would permanently live, she hoped he'd be able to start his new life soon, and wished him well for the future.

I gave my report next. Clearly, much had happened since Oskar's last review in August and I gave a résumé, concentrating on the positives, including gym and swimming, which he still loved. I mentioned CAMHS, and how contact was going with his brother, his aunt and her family, which was obviously important.

'And contact with his mother?' the IRO asked.

'It's just two days a week and generally it's about the same.'

'Thank you,' the IRO said. 'I assume you'll keep in touch with Oskar after he leaves?'

'Oh yes, for as long as he wants to.'

'Will you still foster?' he asked, which had nothing to do with the review and surprised me a little.

'Yes, why?' I asked.

'I just wondered if you were thinking of retiring. You've been fostering a long time.'

I smiled. 'No, I've no plans to retire yet.'

'Good,' Elaine said.

Andrew went next and began by talking about the outcome of the court hearing, the legal complexities of Oskar's case – a child in care going to live in another country. He said his visit to Dol and Ivan had gone well and their assessment was nearly complete, and that he'd visited the school Oskar would be attending, which I already knew. He said that phone contact between Oskar and his mother had been stopped in preparation for the move, and he was hoping that would take place at the end of November or early December. Once he'd finished his report, the IRO read out a short report from CAMHS, which basically said that Oskar was only part way through the therapy and needed more.

'Will Oskar receive therapy after the move?' the IRO asked Andrew.

'That's one of the issues I'm looking into,' Andrew said. 'There is no direct equivalent of CAMHS in Oskar's home country, but we may be able to fund some private therapy if necessary. Dol and Ivan are very practical, down-to-earth people and feel that once Oskar has settled in with them the bad things that happened to him here will fade and he won't need therapy, but the offer is there.'

Edith went next and said much the same as she usually did: that her role was to supervise, support and monitor me in all aspects of fostering, she visited regularly and was satisfied I was providing a good standard of care for Oskar. The IRO thanked her. There was nothing from Roksana, so the IRO asked Elaine Summer to fetch Oskar. Five minutes later he came into the room with her and slid shyly into the seat next to me.

'Welcome, Oskar,' the IRO said, and then asked him about school, swimming, gym and Leo. He replied with short answers in a small voice, occasionally glancing up at us self-consciously.

'Thank you for filling in your review form. Shall I read it out?' the IRO asked.

'No, thank you,' Oskar replied politely, and the IRO smiled.

'Do you have any questions?' he asked him.

Oskar shook his head.

'This will probably be your last review. Do you know why?'

'Because I'm leaving,' Oskar said. 'But I don't mind. I don't really like these reviews.'

We all laughed. Well done, Oskar, I thought.

The IRO closed the meeting just as the klaxon sounded for the end of school. Elaine Summer said she needed to leave smartish and offered to take Oskar to his class.

'Thank you for attending his review,' the IRO said. 'And allowing us to use your office. You'll be sent a copy of the minutes. I'll set a date for the next review, although I'm hoping it won't be necessary.'

I hoped so too, for if we did have another review it would mean Oskar would still be in care three months after he should have been starting his new life abroad with his forever family.

CHAPTER TWENTY-EIGHT

LEAVING

It hadn't escaped my notice that Andrew had told the review he was aiming to move Oskar towards the end of November or early December. He'd previously said the middle to end of November, so the timescale had already slipped back. While my family and I were more than happy to look after Oskar for as long as necessary, he was in no man's land, with one foot in each home, and country, which of course was very unsettling. Every Skype call to his brother, aunt and family strengthened his bond with them as he got to know them better and learnt more about the life he would be living with them. But he also had a bond with us and his mother, so when he saw her he came away feeling guilty and confused. He began telling her and me and my family he loved us many times a day, which was heart-wrenching. I talked to him about his feelings and reassured him.

I didn't hear from Andrew again until the third week in November. I knew there'd be a lot going on behind the scenes. When he phoned, I was hoping he had the news we'd been waiting for – Oskar's departure date. But having asked how Oskar was, Andrew said he was aiming to have Oskar home by Christmas, but it wasn't guaranteed! My heart fell for Oskar. There were some outstanding formalities that he didn't go into. He also said he'd spoken to Dol and asked her if she would be able to fly out and collect Oskar when the time came, but she couldn't leave Luka, so he would take Oskar home. He asked me to tell Oskar he was doing his best to have him home by Christmas and he'd be in touch as soon as he had a definite date.

I told Oskar that afternoon when he came out of school and he was angry – with me and Andrew. He stamped his foot and said he hated us both, which was understandable. Then the following day at contact he became angry with his mother. 'I don't know what's got into him!' Roksana declared when I collected him. 'He wasn't like this when he lived with me.' Suggesting I was responsible for his bad behaviour. I explained that Oskar was feeling very confused and frustrated by the delay.

'Well, he doesn't have to take it out on me,' she said.

The contact supervisor was still there writing – a pointless exercise, I thought, as Oskar's case had been to court and a decision had been made.

I continued with our routine and kept Oskar's life as normal as possible as November rolled into December. I began Christmas shopping and bought presents for Oskar. If he did leave before Christmas, he would take them with him. The following weekend we put up our Christmas decorations and when we Skyped Dol, Oskar pointed them out in our front room with a mixture of joy and sadness. 'I am always with you at Christmas,' he said, 'but Andrew says I might not be this year.' Which was true. He and his mother had always gone home for Christmas; indeed, it was the only time Oskar did go, as far as I knew.

'That's because when you come home this time it will be for good,' Dol said positively. 'Try to be patient.'

'But I want to be there for this Christmas!' Oskar scowled.

'That's a funny face,' Dol said. 'I prefer the happy one.'

He spoke to Luka and the rest of the family, and of course the children were excited and looking forward to Christmas. They chatted about what happened in their house, which didn't help Oskar, as he might not be there.

Finally, on 7 December, when I was thinking Oskar would almost certainly be with us for Christmas, Andrew phoned. 'News at last,' he said, and I held my breath. 'I'm booking the flights for Thursday the fourteenth.'

'Thank goodness,' I sighed. 'Oskar will be pleased.'

'I'll let you know the time once I've confirmed the flight. The last contact with his mother will be this Thursday. I'll be there while they say goodbye. Roksana won't fly out until Christmas Eve.'

Oskar was elated when I told him after school that day, and then he looked sad. 'I'll miss you,' he said, and wanted a big hug.

'We'll miss you too,' I said. 'But we'll speak on the phone.'

'I'll see Mummy at Christmas, but I won't see you,' he said, clearly having thought about it.

'I'll ask your Aunty Dol if we can Skype at Christmas so we can all see each other,' I suggested. It helped and he looked less sad.

Oskar told Adrian, Lucy and Paula he was going very soon as they came home, and of course they had mixed feelings. They were pleased for him, even though they had quietly been hoping – as I had – that he would be with us for Christmas. But as adults who had been fostering for years, they knew what to say so that Oskar remained positive.

The following morning in the school playground he told Leo he was going home. I asked Leo's mother Julia to keep 13

December free, as I would give Oskar his leaving party straight after school. I also gave her Dol's phone number and said Dol had hers so Leo and Oskar could keep in touch.

The final contact loomed. I knew from experience just how upsetting it could be: that moment when the child and their parents have to say goodbye forever, or at least until the child is an adult and can decide for themselves if they wish to see their parent. But that's a lifetime away, and final contacts are unbelievably heart-breaking. I still carry the memories of some parting scenes from years ago, as vivid and emotional now as they were at the time. When I think of them my eyes fill.

However, Oskar's last contact wasn't as upsetting as it might have been, because he was seeing his mother again at Christmas – only two weeks away. I thought the real upset would come when she left him in the New Year with no plans to return for many months. Andrew was there when I collected Oskar at the end of contact and watched as Roksana and Oskar said their goodbyes. It's usual for the social worker to be present. 'I'm so happy we're going home for Christmas,' Oskar said as he hugged his mother goodbye.

'So am I,' she replied and, drawing back, kissed his forehead. And that was it. Oskar came to my side.

I said goodbye to Roksana, wished her well for the future and gave her the Christmas present and card I'd bought. She looked surprised, thanked me and then thanked me for taking care of Oskar, so we parted on good terms. She and Andrew stayed in the room while Oskar and I left.

'I'll miss Mummy,' Oskar said on our way out. 'But I'll see her again in two weeks.'

* * *

Far more upsetting was Oskar saying goodbye to my mother. It wasn't possible for Mum to come to Oskar's leaving party, so the following Saturday – the last before Oskar left – I took him to see her straight after gym. Paula came with me. I knew it was going to be emotional, for this really would be goodbye. As soon as we entered Mum's home, Oskar threw his arms around her and, burying his face in her, cried, 'I'm going to miss you so much, Nana.'

Mum immediately teared up, which of course upset Paula and me. We can't bear to see her unhappy.

'I don't suppose I'll see you again at my age,' she said, her voice thick with emotion. Which upset Paula and me even more.

'Please don't say that, Nana,' Paula said, taking a tissue from her pocket.

'I'm not getting any younger, love.'

I swallowed my emotion and tried to stay positive. 'Mum, we're hoping to Skype Oskar at Christmas,' I said. 'You'll be with us for Christmas, so you'll be able to see and talk to him then.'

'I hope so,' she said bravely, and, taking Oskar's hand, she took him into the living room. Paula and I followed, our hearts going out to Mum.

She and Oskar sat quietly together on the sofa, holding hands and gazing down the garden for some moments as little birds came to the feeder. Mum then picked up one of the story books she had set out ready on the coffee table and began to read from one of his favourites. She keeps books and toys at her house just for the children we foster. She (and Dad when he was alive) always made such a fuss of the children we looked after, and bonded with them. Mum had grown especially close to Oskar, I think because of his age, what he had been through and because we'd seen her most weekends. She once confided in me that Oskar reminded her of Adrian in some ways. I knew what she meant. It wasn't so much his physical appearance, although Adrian did have similar hair colouring at Oskar's age; it was their mannerisms, facial expressions and cheeky smile – just like Adrian had at that age.

When Mum had finished reading and she and Oskar seemed a bit brighter, I suggested we go out for lunch as planned. It was very subdued.

'Will you have food like this when you live with your aunt?' Mum asked Oskar, trying to make conversation.

'I don't know,' Oskar replied.

'It will be nice for you to live with your brother,' Paula said positively.

'Yes,' Oskar said unenthusiastically.

'You'll be fine once you're there,' I told him.

Mum ate very little and I thought that maybe I shouldn't have brought Oskar to say goodbye and phoned instead.

Later, when it was time to go, I said quietly to Mum that we would keep the goodbyes short. She'd bought Oskar a card and present, which was kind of her. Oskar's eyes glistened with tears as she gave them to him.

'Thank you, Nana. I love you,' he said, and wrapped his arms tightly around her.

It was the first time he'd told her he loved her, although he'd heard us say it – when we said goodbye either in person or on the phone. It was something we always did, unlike his mother.

'I love you too, dear,' Mum said. 'You're a good boy. Thank you for coming into my life.'

Paula looked closed to tears and I was struggling. 'We'll be off now then, Mum,' I said, my voice catching. 'We'll phone you once we're home.'

'Yes, love. Take care. Love you.'

'Love you too. You stay indoors,' I told her. 'It's cold outside.' She liked to wave us off at the door, but I could see how upset everyone was getting. 'I'll phone you once we're home.' With a final goodbye, we went out and I drew the door to behind me, leaving Mum in the hall.

'I don't want to go,' Oskar said as we got in the car.

'I know, love.'

Paula sat with him in the back as I drove. After about ten minutes I was so worried about Mum that I asked Paula to phone her and make sure she was all right. The first time she tried it went through to answerphone, which worried me even more. Then a few minutes later she tried again and Mum answered.

'Nana, it's Paula. Mum's driving. Are you OK?'

Paula listened and said, 'All right, I'll tell her. Speak soon. Love you.' Then to me, she said, 'Nana says she's OK, but she's going to have an early night so not to phone her when we get home.'

Which I had to accept, although it did nothing to alleviate my concern for her. She frets and worries about the children we look after just as much as we do. I think as she's got older she finds it more difficult to cope with suffering in the world and saying goodbye. Her words about not seeing Oskar again at her age were an uncomfortable reminder she wouldn't be with us forever, which was heart-breaking. I couldn't bear to think of a time when we wouldn't have Mum, and neither could my children. She'd been there for us all with her love and compassion, in good times and bad.

I respected Mum's request not to phone her when we got home, so I phoned her first thing in the morning. She was always up early, even on a Sunday, and she'd just come in from topping up the bird feeder and sounded brighter. 'The birds are so hungry at this time of year,' she said. 'Sorry about yesterday. Is Oskar all right?'

'Yes. Thanks for the present. He opened it in the car. He'll treasure that forever.' It was a silver money box in the shape of a bear. Mum knew he liked his teddy bear – he'd shown her Luka. She'd bought Adrian, Lucy and Paula silver money boxes when they'd been little, so it showed the level of her affection for Oskar.

'A little keepsake to remember me by,' she said.

'It's lovely, Mum, very thoughtful of you. I'll be over to see you next weekend as usual.'

'Good. I'll look forward to it. Love you.'

'Love you too, Mum.'

Andrew emailed the details of Oskar's departure. Their flight was at 2.30 p.m. on Thursday and he would collect Oskar at 10.30. He had paid for extra luggage, so Oskar could have three bags in the hold with a weight of 32kg each. Andrew knew how important it was that Oskar took everything with him. Not only would it mean that Dol wouldn't have to start buying new, but his belongings were part of Oskar's history. Three suitcases might sound like a lot, but as well as his clothes he had all his toys and the Christmas presents we'd bought for him. I replied to Andrew that I'd make sure the bags were within the limit and would have Oskar ready by 10.30 a.m. I said I wasn't planning on taking Oskar to art therapy on Wednesday, as it was his last day at school and I was giving him a little leaving party straight afterwards – from 4.30 till 6.30 – which I hoped Andrew would be able to come to. He emailed back thanking me for the invitation and saying he'd look in, and that it was fine for Oskar not to go to therapy.

I arranged with Dol to Skype on Tuesday evening rather than Wednesday because of Oskar's leaving do. He and his family were so excited – in forty-eight hours he'd be with them. Ivan was at work, but Luka told us that Oskar's bedroom was nearly finished, and if it wasn't, he could share his room. Their dog barked in the background, seeming to confirm this. Dol told Oskar that he would go to school the following week for the last few days of term before they broke up for Christmas, which would get him used to it ready for the new term.

Oskar groaned as many six-year-olds would do at the prospect of a new school term, and then asked, 'Will my social worker be staying with us?'

'No,' Dol replied. 'Andrew is going to bring you here on Thursday and will stay in a bed and breakfast on Thursday night. He's going to visit us on Friday, and then fly home that evening. He'll return for one last visit in the New Year, and if everything is all right we won't see him again.'

'Good. I don't mind not seeing him any more,' Oskar said, and I saw Dol smile.

Dol said she'd text me to confirm that Oskar had arrived safely and we'd Skype at Christmas and then stay in touch. I thanked her and said if she needed any help at all in connection with Oskar she could call me. I didn't doubt her ability to parent Oskar, but it occurred to me that she'd only really seen him at Christmas for the last few years, so I probably knew him better than she did at present.

Oskar was very excited after the call and it took a long time for him to settle and go to sleep. He'd only mentioned his mother once since their final contact and that was simply to say he'd be seeing her at Christmas.

The next morning, Oskar's last at school, Leo and the other

300

children in their class ran over to greet him as soon as we entered the playground. They were excited for him and told him he was lucky to be going on a plane to live in another country. They made such a fuss of him and I thought back to the solitary child I'd first stood with in the playground, withdrawn and miserable from the secret of abuse. When it was time for school to start, I wished him a nice day and waited while he went in.

When he came out at the end of school, he was carrying the biggest leaving card I've ever seen. Made by the children in his class, on the front was a large photograph of them all, with Mrs Williams, Elaine Summer and Miss Jordan. Inside, everyone had signed it. It was a lovely gesture and I knew Oskar would treasure it. To shouts of goodbye and good luck, we left the playground and I helped Oskar carry the card to the car. Once home, I stood it with his other leaving cards on the table, where I laid out the buffet for his leaving party.

On the invitations I'd set the time of the party as 4.30 till 6.30 to allow the children he'd invited from his class a chance to go home and change out of their school uniforms. Oskar changed into casual clothes too, and at dead on 4.30 p.m. the doorbell rang. Oskar flew to answer it and first to arrive was Leo, with his mother and older brother. They gave Oskar a card and present and I reminded him to say thank you. Next to arrive was Paula, home from college; Lucy and Adrian would come as soon as they could after work. Miss Jordan, Mrs Williams and Elaine Summer arrived together, followed by a succession of six children who Oskar had become friends with, and their mothers. I couldn't invite the whole class, so Oskar had chosen his closest friends. Everyone had brought a card and present. 'It's like Christmas!' Oskar declared excitedly.

Lucy and Adrian arrived just after five o'clock, quickly changed out of their work clothes and joined us downstairs for the buffet and drinks. Paula and I arranged some games and made sure all the children won a little prize. Andrew arrived for the last half-hour, but Edith didn't make it. I assumed something must have come up, but Oskar didn't miss her. I was touched that so many had come to wish Oskar all the best for the future. He was so happy; even when it was time to say goodbye his mood didn't drop. But I thought it might be very different the following morning when the house was quiet and there was just him and me to say good-bye. That's when it would hit us both.

CHAPTER TWENTY-NINE

UNEXPECTED NEWS

Adrian, Lucy and Paula said goodbye to Oskar as they left the following morning. They knew it was important to stay upbeat and positive, despite what they might be feeling. Adrian gave Oskar a high five as he said goodbye and told him that Kirsty sent her best wishes too. Paula put on a brave smile as she hugged Oskar goodbye, but Lucy went very pale, so much so that I asked her if she was feeling all right.

'Not really,' she said, but then she left for work without saying anything further. I assumed it was because she was having to say goodbye to Oskar. It often affected her deeply when children left, as she knew what it was like to have to move, from when she'd been in care herself before coming to live with me.

By 9.15 a.m. there was just Oskar and me, with Sammy asleep by the radiator in the living room. The house was silent and seemed to have fallen sad too. Oskar had eaten a little breakfast, but not much, and asked if he could watch television. I thought that was a good idea, so after he'd brushed his teeth he watched a children's programme while I put away the last of his belongings. I dragged all the cases downstairs and lined them up in the hall, then checked the house for any stray items, and joined Oskar in the living room. I sat on the sofa and held his hand. He was wearing the watch we'd bought him as a leaving present.

'I've enjoyed looking after you,' I said. 'We'll all miss you, but I know you'll be happy with your family. You're a good boy.'

He didn't reply but snuggled in close, resting his head on my shoulder. Sometimes silence and a small gesture can speak volumes. I continued to sit beside him, gazing, unseeing, at the television, and making the most of our last few minutes together. I'm not sure he was really interested in the programme either, but it was a distraction for him as it was for me. At 10.15 I told him to go to the toilet so he was ready for when Andrew arrived. As he returned downstairs the doorbell rang. 'That'll be Andrew,' I said, going to answer it. Oskar's eyes filled.

'I wish you were coming with me,' he cried, and wrapped his arms around me so tightly I couldn't move. I hugged him for a moment and then opened the front door.

'Are you OK?' Andrew asked, for clearly we weren't.

'Oskar's ready,' I said stoically.

'Excellent.' He smiled reassuringly.

Andrew's car was parked right outside, and I helped Oskar in as Andrew loaded the cases. Then it was time for me to say goodbye. Oskar was sitting, head down and seatbelt on. I leant in. 'Bye, love.'

'I love you, Cathy.'

'I love you too.' I kissed his cheek. 'We'll Skype at Christmas and you can tell me all about what you've been up to. Bye, love.' I closed his car door.

'Thanks for looking after him,' Andrew said.

'It was a pleasure.'

I stood on the pavement, my face set to a smile, and waved Oskar off. Once they were out of sight, I returned indoors.

The Christmas decorations stirred in the draught from the closing door. Sammy had left the comfort of the radiator and, sensing something was going on, had come into the hall to find out what.

'Oskar's left,' I said, and picked him up. I carried him through to the living room, where I sat on the sofa and stroked his soft, silky fur as he purred. I find something comforting in stroking a cat, and Sammy seemed pleased too. 'Oskar's gone to start his new life,' I told him. 'I wonder who we will be looking after next.' He purred an acknowledgement.

I didn't have to wonder long, for five minutes later, while I was still sitting on the sofa and thinking of Oskar, the land-line rang. I reached out and picked up the handset. It was Edith. 'Sorry I couldn't make Oskar's leaving party,' she said. 'Has he gone now?'

'Yes, about ten minutes ago.'

'We've had a referral for a fourteen-year-old girl who we need to move quickly. She's very angry with –' But as Edith began giving me her details, I heard the front door open and close. I wasn't expecting anyone home, and for a moment I thought Oskar had returned, which was ridiculous, as he didn't have a key and was on his way to the airport. Sammy had also heard the door and pricked up his ears.

Familiar footsteps came down the hall and Lucy appeared in the living room. 'I need to talk to you,' she said seriously, clearly upset.

'Edith, I'm sorry, I'll have to get back to you.' I ended the call.

'What's the matter, love?' I asked, worried, and went to her.

'Mum, I'm so sorry,' she said. Her face crumpled and she fell into my arms.

'What is it? Have you lost your job?' I asked anxiously as I held her. It seemed the most likely explanation for her suddenly appearing in the day.

'No, I've taken time off work. I've been to see a doctor.'

Fear gripped me. 'Why? Are you ill?'

'No. Please don't be angry with me,' she sobbed.

'I won't. But tell me what's the matter, please.'

Another small sob and then she said, 'I'm pregnant and I don't know what to do.'

At that point, neither did I.

But this story is about Oskar, and I need to finish it first.

On Thursday evening Dol texted to say Oskar had arrived safely but was very tired. We gave him time to settle in, and then on Christmas Day evening we Skyped. Not for long, as they were busy with their Christmas, as we were with ours, but long enough for us all – including my mother – to see Oskar was happy with his new family. Roksana was there in the background and called hello. The children talked excitedly about their presents and then we all wished each other a Merry Christmas and said we'd chat again in the New Year. Dol and I had already agreed that it was best if we took our cue from Oskar and Skyped when he wanted to. I knew from experience that often children wanted to keep in touch regularly with their carer to begin with, but then as they moved on with their lives it tailed off and sometimes stopped completely. It would be Oskar's decision. Some children keep in touch and some make contact again after a long gap, which is a lovely surprise. Foster carers are always pleased to hear from the children they've looked after.

* * *

If it hadn't been for Dol, I probably wouldn't have found out the result of the criminal court case against Oskar's abusers. Once a child leaves, the foster carer is very rarely updated by the social services. In March, just after Andrew's final visit, Dol told me that both men had been found guilty and were now serving prison sentences, which was a great relief to us all. Andrew had also told Dol there was another man living in the house who was wanted by the police, though it wasn't Mr Nowak.

'Roksana was far too trusting,' Dol said to me. 'In those types of houses you end up living with strangers. It's no place for a child.'

I agreed. 'Thankfully Oskar's got you and that's all behind him now,' I said. There was just Dol and me on Skype now, as Oskar had finished talking and gone off to play. 'Dol, there's something I'd like to ask you. I've been thinking about it for a while. And please don't take offence.'

'I won't,' she said uncertainly. 'What is it?'

'During the months we've been Skyping, I couldn't help but notice the state of Luka's wheelchair. It seems old and difficult for him to manoeuvre, especially outside.'

She gave a small, rueful laugh. 'Yes, I know. It was worn out when we got it years ago. It was donated by a charity so we can't complain.'

'Dol, if you and Ivan agree, I'd like to buy Luka a new wheelchair.'

'No, you can't do that,' she exclaimed. 'Of course not.'

'I'd like to, really. It would make me very happy. But only if it's OK with you, Ivan and Luka.' Her eyes filled, which choked me up. I hadn't intended to upset her. 'Please say yes,' I added.

'Luka would love a new wheelchair,' she said, wiping away a tear. 'Of course he would. He doesn't complain, but it's very uncomfortable for him, and we can't afford to replace it. Yes, I agree, that would be wonderful for him, and I know Ivan will think so too. I'll say yes, if you're sure.'

'I am. Fantastic. Shall I arrange to have the wheelchair sent to you?' I asked. 'Or send you the money so you can buy it?'

'I don't mind, although we don't have a shop like that anywhere near us. We'll need to find one, when Ivan has the time.'

'I've done some research online and I could order it and have it delivered to you. Would that be easier?' I asked.

'Oh yes, much easier, thank you. I don't know what to say.'

'Nothing. I'm pleased I can help a little. You do so much for the boys. They are very lucky to have you.'

She teared up again as we said goodbye and I felt emotional too. They were a lovely family who didn't have much and I was delighted to be able to do something to help. I immediately went online and ordered the motorized wheelchair I'd had my eye on. I'd already spent some time researching them and this was one of the best available. The retail outlet that sold them was over a hundred kilometres from where Dol lived, but they delivered and offered an aftersales service with an extended warranty.

Four days later Dol texted to say the wheelchair had arrived and Luka wanted to Skype. I went to my computer in the front room and the call came through. There was Luka, sitting proudly in his new wheelchair. 'Hi, Aunty Cathy! Look at me!'

I smiled. Dol was holding up her phone with the camera pointing towards Luka so I could see him as he moved forwards, backwards and in circles, showing me what the wheelchair could do. We went around the downstairs, out across the yard, then in again. I was pleased to see that it glided effortlessly over the ground, giving him a freedom he'd never had before. Smiling from ear to ear, Luka finally drew the wheelchair to a halt and looked at me in earnest. 'Cathy, thank you so very much. You've no idea what this means to me.'

I think I did.

And what of Lucy and her predicament, and the angry fourteen-year-old Edith wanted me to foster? Well, that's another story and I'll save it for my next book. Thank you for joining me on Oskar's journey. For the latest on him and the other children in my books, please visit www.cathyglass.co.uk.

SUGGESTED TOPICS FOR
READING-GROUP DISCUSSION

Bearing in mind Roksana's situation, what changes could she have made to give her a better chance of having Oskar returned to her care?

What are the advantages and disadvantages of multiple-occupancy living? Could it ever be suitable for a child?

What are the early signs that Oskar might have been sexually abused?

How would you describe Roksana's character and her relationship with her sons? How much sympathy do you have for her?

Describe Edith's role as Cathy's supervising social worker. How might Edith improve her role?

School is safe and offers continuity for a child in care. Discuss.

What is the purpose of regular reviews for children in care? How effective do you think they are? How might they be improved?

Like many of Cathy's previous foster children, Oskar forms a strong bond with her mother, Nana. Why do you think this might be?

Cathy believes it is the right decision for Oskar to live permanently with his aunt. Do you agree? What problems, if any, might he face once he's moved?

At the end of the book, Lucy delivers some life-changing news, which Cathy puts on hold in order to finish Oskar's story. Write the first paragraph of the next book.

Cathy Glass

———

One remarkable woman, more than **150** foster children cared for.

Cathy Glass has been a foster carer for twenty-five years, during which time she has looked after more than 150 children, as well as raising three children of her own. She was awarded a degree in education and psychology as a mature student, and writes under a pseudonym. To find out more about Cathy and her story visit **www.cathyglass.co.uk**.

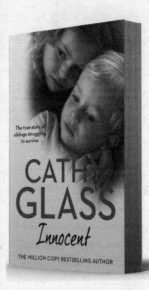

Innocent

Siblings Molly and Kit arrive at Cathy's frightened, injured and ill

The parents say they are not to blame. Could the social services have got it wrong?

Finding Stevie

Fourteen-year-old Stevie is exploring his gender identity

Like many young people, he spends time online, but Cathy is shocked when she learns his terrible secret.

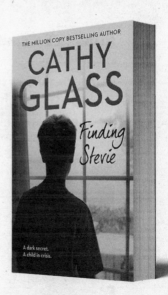

Where Has Mummy Gone?

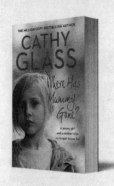

When Melody is taken into care, she fears her mother won't cope alone

It is only when Melody's mother vanishes that what has really been going on at home comes to light.

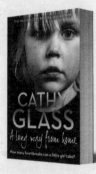

A Long Way from Home

Abandoned in an orphanage, Anna's future looks bleak until she is adopted

Anna's new parents love her, so why does she end up in foster care?

Cruel to be Kind

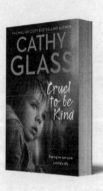

Max is shockingly overweight and struggles to make friends

Cathy faces a challenge to help this unhappy boy.

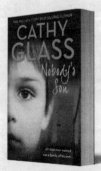

Nobody's Son

Born in prison and brought up in care, Alex has only ever known rejection

He is longing for a family of his own, but again the system fails him.

Can I Let You Go?

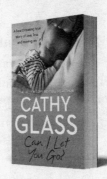

Faye is 24, pregnant and has learning difficulties as a result of her mother's alcoholism

Can Cathy help Faye learn enough to parent her child?

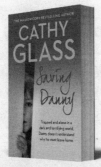

The Silent Cry

A mother battling depression. A family in denial

Cathy is desperate to help before something terrible happens.

Girl Alone

An angry, traumatized young girl on a path to self-destruction

Can Cathy discover the truth behind Joss's dangerous behaviour before it's too late?

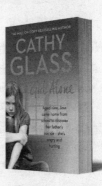

Saving Danny

Danny's parents can no longer cope with his challenging behaviour

Calling on all her expertise, Cathy discovers a frightened little boy who just wants to be loved.

The Child Bride

A girl blamed and abused for dishonouring her community

Cathy discovers the devastating truth.

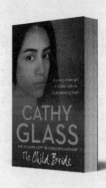

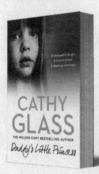

Daddy's Little Princess

A sweet-natured girl with a complicated past

Cathy picks up the pieces after events take a dramatic turn.

Will You Love Me?

A broken child desperate for a loving home

The true story of Cathy's adopted daughter Lucy.

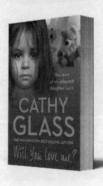

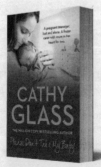

Please Don't Take My Baby

Seventeen-year-old Jade is pregnant, homeless and alone

Cathy has room in her heart for two.

Another Forgotten Child

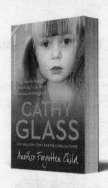

Eight-year-old Aimee was on the child-protection register at birth

Cathy is determined to give her the happy home she deserves.

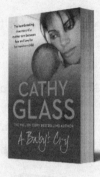

A Baby's Cry

A newborn, only hours old, taken into care

Cathy protects tiny Harrison from the potentially fatal secrets that surround his existence.

The Night the Angels Came

A little boy on the brink of bereavement

Cathy and her family make sure Michael is never alone.

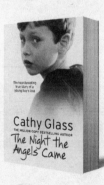

Mummy Told Me Not to Tell

A troubled boy sworn to secrecy

After his dark past has been revealed, Cathy helps Reece to rebuild his life.

I Miss Mummy

Four-year-old Alice doesn't understand why she's in care

Cathy fights for her to have the happy home she deserves.

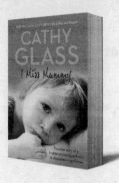

The Saddest Girl in the World

A haunted child who refuses to speak

Do Donna's scars run too deep for Cathy to help?

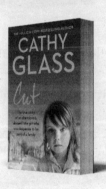

Cut

Dawn is desperate to be loved

Abused and abandoned, this vulnerable child pushes Cathy and her family to their limits.

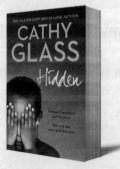

Hidden

The boy with no past

Can Cathy help Tayo to feel like he belongs again?

Damaged

A forgotten child

Cathy is Jodie's last hope. For the first time, this abused young girl has found someone she can trust.

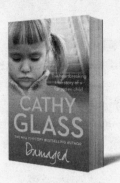

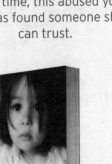

Run, Mummy, Run

The gripping story of a woman caught in a horrific cycle of abuse, and the desperate measures she must take to escape.

My Dad's a Policeman

The dramatic short story about a young boy's desperate bid to keep his family together.

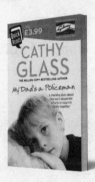

The Girl in the Mirror

Trying to piece together her past, Mandy uncovers a dreadful family secret that has been blanked from her memory for years.

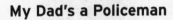

About Writing
and How to Publish

A clear, concise practical
guide on writing and the best
ways to get published.

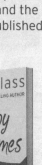

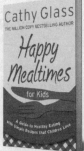

Happy Mealtimes
for Kids

A guide to healthy eating
with simple recipes that
children love.

Happy Adults

A practical guide to achieving lasting
happiness, contentment and success.
The essential manual for getting
the best out of life.

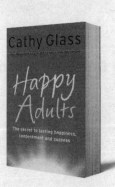

Happy Kids

A clear and concise guide to
raising confident, well-behaved
and happy children.

CATHY GLASS WRITING AS
LISA STONE

www.lisastonebooks.co.uk

The new crime thrillers that will chill you to the bone . . .

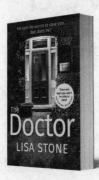

THE DOCTOR

How much do you know about the couple next door?

STALKER

Security cameras are there to keep us safe. Aren't they?

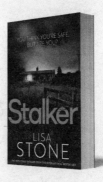

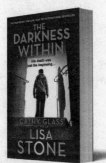

THE DARKNESS WITHIN

You know your son better than anyone. Don't you?

Be amazed
Be moved
Be inspired

Follow Cathy:

/cathy.glass.180

@CathyGlassUK

www.cathyglass.co.uk